FROM ANCIENT ORIGINS TO POETIC REVELATIONS

by

Laura Jones

Abstract

This thesis compares depictions of yoga in literature with the practices and philosophies described in yoga treatises between 400 BCE and 1500 CE. This comparison, while broad, will help establish a basis for future research into the pre-modern public perception of yoga and yogis, as well as provide some insight into how yoga evolved and was received both in the exogenous and endogenous spheres. This study employs a mixed-methods approach combining intellectual history, adaptive reuse, and intertextuality studies. It begins by examining yoga and philosophy treatises that provide the basis for various popular schools of yoga. The second section looks at early Islamicate engagements with yoga. The final section analyzes depictions of yoga in Sanskrit literature.

The primary findings indicate that non-yoga practitioners in premodern South Asia were both curious about yoga while also wary of its claims to unlock magical powers in dedicated practitioners. There seemed to be a public awareness of what yoga was and who practiced it, but until the early-medieval period, circa seventh century CE, it was not recognized as a homogenous school. While the depictions of yogis all represented ascetics, the actual practices, abilities, and beliefs themselves diverged drastically, and whether it was accepted as a legitimate set of practices seemed to depend on the author more than their background.

These results suggest that there was never any single definition of yoga, nor a broadly recognized school of yoga. Rather, there was an array of people who practiced asceticism and operated on the peripheries of the established religious traditions. The literary responses were initially curious. Yoga became more formalized in the second millennia and adopted more transgressive practices, and the writers were more cautious about the schools, often depicting them as blasphemous. Around 1500 CE we see more acceptance of yoga practices by writers.

Table of Contents

List of Tables

List of Figures

Introduction

This thesis is focused on depictions of yoga in premodern South Asian literature. Drawing on theories from intellectual history and cultural anthropology, I explore how people across time in South Asia viewed the practices and practitioners of yoga. I also examine why they may have been depicted as they were and assess what their depiction tells us about the writers and the practices themselves. Following a new historical methodology of reading *kāvya* poets as actively participating within the intellectual history that they find themselves in,[1] as well as utilizing the theoretical framework of adaptive reuse,[2] I study prominent instances within early Islamicate engagements with yoga and Sanskrit courtly poetry and theatre where poets have engaged in ornate depictions of practical yoga and philosophical yoga. This thesis aims not to make new claims about the origins of yoga—which other scholars have analyzed in detail—or to situate yoga practices within any one tradition but rather to examine how yoga was viewed outside the formal corpus.

In the first section, I reference Sanskrit yoga treatises, including the *Bhagavad Gītā* (c. 300 BCE),[3] which is the first text wherein yoga is used to describe a defined set of practices; the *Vaiśeṣika Sūtra* (c. 100 CE),[4] which helps lay out the philosophical basis of yoga; *Pātañjala Yogaśāstra* (c. 350 CE),[5] which is the first time yoga is treated as its own school of thought and

---

[1] Adheesh Sathaye, "Total Absorption: Locating Kālidāsa in the Intellectual History of Rasa," in *Kālidāsa's Nāyikās*, ed. Harsha Dehejia (Delhi: DK Printworld, 2019), 37-53.
[2] Elisa Freschi and Philipp A. Maas, ed. *Adaptive Reuse: Aspects of Creativity in South Asian Cultural History* (Germany: Deutsche Morgenländische Gesellschaft, 2017).
[3] Laurie L. Patton, *The Bhagavad Gita* (England: Penguin Classics, 2008).
[4] Śaśiprabhā Kumār, *Classical Vaiśeṣika in Indian philosophy: On Knowing and What is to be Known* (London: Routledge, 2013).
[5] Rāma Prasāda, trans., *Patañjali's Yoga Sutras: With the Commentary of Vyāsa and the Gloss of Vāchaspati Miśra* (New Delhi: Munshiram Manoharlal Publishers Private Ltd., 1974).

practice;[6] the *Sāṁkhyakārikā* (c. 200 CE),[7] which provides the basis of the philosophy that yoga practice is built upon; the *Amṛtasiddhi* (c. 1000 CE),[8] which marks a major turning point as the first text to formally incorporate tantric practices, thus setting the foundation for *haṭha* yoga as we know it; the *Yogavāsiṣṭha* (c. 1100 CE),[9] which further develops the philosophical basis for yoga as a nondualist practice*;* and the *Haṭhayogapradīpikā* (c. 1400 CE),[10] which is the earliest extant comprehensive treatise on haṭha yoga. These texts work together to outline the intellectual history within which Kālidāsa and other Sanskrit poets were operating. In section two, I start to examine a wider lens of four Islamicate texts that talk about yogis and yoga practice, including al-Bīrūni's *Kitāb Bātanjal* (c. 1000 CE), an Arabic translation of *Patāñjali's Yogasūtras;* "Medieval Sufi Tales of Jogis," a collection of short stories written by Sufis about yogis (c. 1300 CE); Muhammad Ghawth Gwaliyari's *Bahr al-hayat* (c. 1400 CE), a Sufi translation of the *Amṛtakuṇḍa*, a lost Sanskrit haṭha yoga text; and Mir Sayyid Manjhan Shattari Rajgiri's *Madhumālatī* (c. 1500 CE), a long Sufi poem that includes descriptions of yoga practice. This literary lens that grapples with "othering" the yogis will help contextualize how yogis and yoga were perceived by non-practitioners so that I can use the framework to help analyze the Sanskrit depictions in section three.[11] Section three examines, through the Sanskrit author's eyes, the

[6] Recent scholarship suggests that the Yogasūtras are actually the same author as the first known commentator, and the collection is called *Patañjala Yogaśāstra.* I will explain in further detail in the PYS section below (1.5), but simply put, I may use both terms interchangeably.
[7] Dr. Har Dutt Sharma, *The Sāṃkhya-Kārikā: Iśvara Kṛṣṇa's Memorable Verses on Sāṃkhya Philosophy with the Commentary of Gauḍapādācārya* (Poona: Oriental Book Agency, 1933).
[8] James Mallinson and Péter-Dániel Szántó, ed. and trans., *The Amṛtasiddhi and Amṛtasiddhimūla: The Earliest Texts of the Haṭhayoga Tradition* (France: Institut Français de Pondichéry, 2021).
[9] Swami Venkatesananda, *Vasiṣṭha's Yoga* (Albany N.Y.: State University of New York Press, 1993). I am using the later, expanded text rather than the original text, which has been critically edited and is known as the Mokṣopāya, and edited by Walter Slaje and his team at Halle.
[10] Swami Svātmārāma, *The Hatha Yoga Pradīpikā.* trans. by Pancham Sinh. (Allahabad: Panini Office, 1915)
[11] I explain the use and framework of "othering" later in this introduction.

extent to which yoga, as a physical and spiritual practice in ancient India, was perceived and how it differed from what was described in philosophical texts, and why that might be.

Philosophy, in the context of this thesis, is used to describe any text that deals with theoretical explanations for the meaning of life, reality as we know it, and explanations for how things are and why they are this way. Religion is used to describe schools of belief and practice that have some kind of recognized tradition, believe in some kind of supernatural or divine power (whether dualist or nondualist), have established explanations of philosophical questions, and/or engage in standard practices or rituals. Many of the texts examined here consider themselves to be religious texts, some philosophical texts, and some poetry or stories; what I have found in my analysis is that these lines are often blurred. Poetry can include philosophy and religion, and some texts that claim to be philosophical often include religious content. For instance, *Pātañjali's Yogasūtras* includes quite a lot of philosophy as it explains the basis of reality and our place in it. It also includes descriptions of a deity—*Īśvara*—so has some religious element to it, and it deals very practically with non-philosophical content when it details actions and practices we can undertake. Later texts, such as the *Haṭhayogapradīpikā* deal almost exclusively with physical practices rather than philosophical concepts.

As part of this textual comparison, I use the term "othering," though not in the Foucauldian sense of situating oneself in a hierarchy, but as a way of categorizing groups of people and systems of belief.[12] Al-Bīrūni is widely recognized (and recognized himself, as we will see in section 2.2) as the first Islamicate scholar to engage with yoga philosophy and texts in a respectful way, for the merit of the texts themselves.[13] He noted that scholars before him either

[12] Michel Foucault, *The Order of Things: An Archaeology of the Human Sciences* (London: Routledge, 1989).
[13] See Audrey Truschke, "Defining the Other: An Intellectual History of Sanskrit Lexicons and Grammars of Persian," *Journal of Indian Philosophy* 40, 2012, 635-668; Nurhanisah Senin, "Understanding the 'other': the case of Al-Biruni (973-1048 AD)," *International Journal of Ethics and Systems* 35, no. 3 (2019): 392-409; Mario Kozah,

dismissed non-Islamic religions, practices, and beliefs entirely, or demeaned them. When he frames yoga philosophy as something "other," he means it in a positive sense, as a recognition of difference between yoga philosophy and Islamic philosophy. He also notes the similarities. He notes that the ideas are blasphemous, according to him, but that there is value in understanding them for the sake of understanding the people that he, and other Islamicate scholars, were encountering. I take the same approach when using the term "other" throughout this thesis. While "othering" is often considered to be the author comparing themselves to someone or something and noting the differences for the sake of proving themselves correct, what I find in the works examined in this thesis is that, more often than not, the othering is happening between various groups of people rather than the author and the target. Othering, in the context of these texts, is more of a curiosity, a recognition of "not-sameness" between distinct groups of people, beliefs, and practices. In a way, it is a matter of recognizing that something is changing, something new is happening, and trying to grapple with it being different than what the author is used to, or what is deemed "correct" or "traditional". To state it differently, the othering is essentially a way of classifying or categorizing groups of people for their beliefs and practices, not necessarily to set up opposition between groups, but to examine them as distinct entities (and sometimes oppositional). So, unless otherwise specified, if I use the term "othering," it is not in a judgmental sense, but as a form of comparison wherein the authors are recognizing some distinction between various groups that may not have been made before.

The Birth of Indology as an Islamic Science: Al-Bīrūnī's Treatise on Yoga Psychology (Brill, 2015); Bruce B. Lawrence, "Al-Bīrūnī's Approach to the Comparative Study of Indian Culture" (*Biruni Symposium*, 1976).

Establishing a Timeline

This thesis will examine a multitude of sources. To position them in time and place, I have created the following chart showing what texts I will be examining and approximately when they were written.

Table 1. Textual timeline

Time	Primary Yoga Treatise	Islamicate Depictions	Kavya Depictions
400 BCE-200 CE	*Bhagavad Gītā*		
100-200 CE	*Vaiśeṣika Sūtra*		
200-300 CE	*Sāṁkhyakārikā*		
300-400 CE	*Yogasūtras of Pātañjali*		*Kumārasambhava*
600-700 CE			*Śiśupālavadha*
1000-1100 CE	*Amṛtasiddhi*	*Kitāb Bātanjal*	*Prabodha Chandrodaya*
900-1300 CE	*Yogavāsiṣṭha*	"Medieval Sufi Tales of Jogis"	*Vetālapañcaviṃśati*
1400 CE	*Haṭhayogapradīpikā*	*Bahr al-hayat*	
1500 CE		*Madhumālatī*	

1 The History of Yoga

1.1 What is Yoga?

Before we can discuss the intellectual history of yoga, we need to define what it is. The most basic translation of "yoga" comes from the Sanskrit verbal root √*yuj*, meaning "yoke" or "unite." Most simply, "yoga" is cognate with the English "yoke," as in yoking a horse to a carriage. Each school of yoga defines it in a slightly different way, which will be evident in each text I analyze below.

Yoga as a practice or philosophical system is complicated to define because there are so many different schools of practice and belief that have emerged over the years. The earliest comprehensive sources we have, such as the *Upaniṣads*, show that yoga started in South Asia as ascetic practices with the goal of attaining samādhi (union) between the *ātman* (individual self) and the *brahman* (cosmic whole), i.e., a state of complete consciousness in which one is free from the confines of the material world. The term was used to describe *any* ascetic, not a particular group of people who considered themselves "yogis." Over time, yoga became more complicated. As yoga practitioners encountered other religions, physical places, politics and cultures, various schools with different types of practices and beliefs branched off. Most broadly, yoga is a religious, philosophical, and physical practice system.

Figure 1. Pashupati Seal

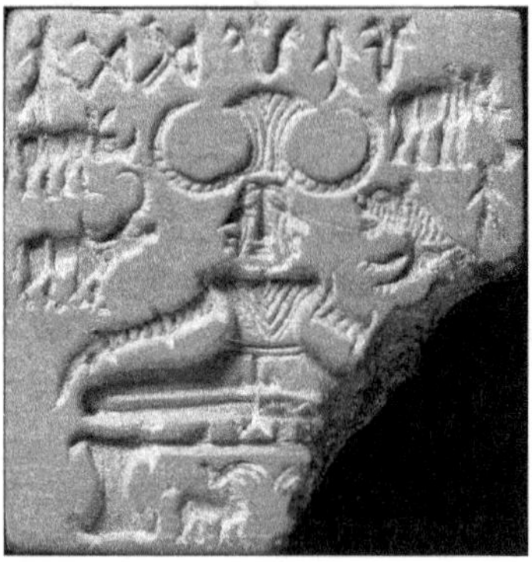

The earliest evidence we have for the practice of yoga is a controversial image of a seated figure on a seal found in the ancient city of Mohenjo-daro in the Indus Valley, circa third millennium BCE. On this seal, known as the Pashupati seal, we see a person seated in a cross-legged pose, wearing a horned headdress, and surrounded by various animals. Various scholars have suggested different interpretations for the imagery on this seal.[14] Regardless of how we interpret this early seal, there is nothing to suggest that yogic practices took place until much later. The term "yogic practices" is meant to encompass a set of techniques that are used for the purpose of uniting the mind and body for the purpose of expanding the ātman to the brahman.

We see evidence of ascetics as early as the *Ṛg Veda*, approximately 1000 BCE, where *munis* (ascetics) are described as having long, streaming hair, being either nude or wearing yellow garments, and able to overcome the limitations of the body.[15] These specific ascetic practices became codified in the Upaniṣads, and what are called *śramaṇa* practices, such as in Buddhism and Jainism, around the sixth and fifth centuries BCE.[16] Contrary to the popular belief maintained by scholars like Georg Feuerstein (2002) that the school of yoga emerged out of the Vedic tradition, yoga as a distinct practice was mentioned first in the Buddhist Yogācāra texts in the first few centuries of the Common Era.[17] It was not until, likely, the third or fourth century CE that the practice of yoga was formalized as its own school in the PYS.[18]

---

[14] Image from unknown Indus Valley Civilization sealmaker from Mohenjodaro archaeological site, Public Domain, https://commons.wikimedia.org/w/index.php?curid=9325528. Since the Indus Valley Civilization that created this seal c. 1900 BCE experienced a demise of its urban culture, we cannot know for sure what this seal is meant to represent, but some scholars such as Marshall have claimed it is an early depiction of the god Śiva who is described in the Śaiva tradition as being an ascetic (Sir J. Marshall, *Mohenjodaro and the Indus Civilization: Being an Official Account of Archaeological Excavations at Mohenjodaro Carried Out by the Government of India Between the Years 1922—2.* (Delhi: Indological Book House, 1931)). However, other scholars, such as Hiltebeitel (1978) and Allchin (1982), have posited other, non-yogic interpretations (see Geoffrey Samuel, *The Origins of Yoga and Tantra: Indic Religions to the Thirteenth Century* (United Kingdom: Cambridge University Press, 2008), 3-4.).

[15] Barbara Stoler Miller, *Yoga: Discipline of Freedom* (New York: Bantam Press, 1998), 8; also see an example in Rg Veda Book 10, Verse 136 as per Ralph T.H. Griffith, *The Hymns of the Rigveda: Translated with a Popular Commentary*, 2nd Edition. (Benares: K.J. Lazarus and Co., 1897), 582.

[16] Samuel, *The Origins of Yoga and Tantra*, 8; Johannes Bronkhorst, *Greater Magadha: Studies in the Culture of Early India* (Leiden: Brill, 2007).

[17] O'Brien-Kop, *Rethinking 'Classical Yoga' and Buddhism*, 163.

[18] Philip A. Maas, "A Concise Historiography of Classical Yoga Philosophy," in *Periodization and Historiography of Indian Philosophy*, ed. Eli Franco (Vienna: De Nobili Research Library, 2013), 66.

It is important to note that not all ascetics are yogis. There were and continue to be people who practiced asceticism all over the world who ascribe to different beliefs and practice for different goals. I will examine in section two one such example of the Sufi orders of Islam, which interacted with yogis and recognized them as similar but somehow different. What differentiates yogis from any other ascetic tradition? Rather than outright disagreeing with the Vedic and Upaniṣadic beliefs, they incorporated many and expanded on others, as we will see in the examination of some primary yoga texts later in this section. Other ascetic practices disavowed the Brahmanical traditions and instead posited opposing viewpoints. Nevertheless, the goals of the ascetic traditions were relatively the same—i.e., to attain spiritual liberation from the physical world.[19] What that meant and how exactly that was to be achieved differed for each ascetic tradition.

Yoga as a codified practice started as a dualistic belief system that treated yoga as a meditative and moral practice intended to achieve liberation from the cycle of rebirth. Over time, while many different schools and practices broke off or began anew by bringing in ideas and practices new to the discipline, there was some unity that remained throughout. One way to narrow down what yoga is and how it was practiced—which is what this thesis will try to do—is to examine texts that call themselves yoga texts. These primary texts claim to be part of a tradition, and many helped spawn adjacent traditions of yogic practices. They described what practices to perform and how to perform them, including how someone should dress, where they should practice, and what they should eat. Secondary texts about yoga, such as Sanskrit and Sufi poetry, also discuss various forms of yoga in unique ways that speak to how yoga was perceived and received by the people writing at the time. While the secondary texts are not telling people

[19] Johannes Bronkhorst. "Systematic Philosophy between the Empires," in *Between the Empires: Society in India 300 BCE to 400 CE*, ed. Patrick Olivelle (New York: Oxford University Press, 2006).

how or what to practice, they are describing the practices and philosophies, as well as the people who are considered (or consider themselves) yogis. Their depictions may not be accurate, and are biased towards the author's beliefs, but they still provide an idea of how yoga practice and philosophy was treated over time by different groups of people. Whether we are examining treatises or poetry, these texts all represent a body of work that constitutes some kind of thread, some unified whole that composed what we recognize as yoga.

1.1.1 Historical Context

Before we can understand how yoga developed, we must understand the context it arose in. Two polarizing metaphysical ideas were prominent in the earliest records of South Asian thought, particularly in the north-west of the subcontinent: (i) the Upaniṣadic idea that there exists a permanent self or soul (ātman) that transmigrates,[20] and (ii) the nihilistic idea that upon death the person completely ceases to be and never transmigrates. As far as records show, the Upaniṣadic idea was far more culturally accepted *en masse*.[21] The two major questions that both lines of thought were trying to answer were: (i) why do we suffer and (ii) how do we end suffering?[22] In order to answer these questions, there seemed to be two polarizing ways of living, either (i) to lavishly enjoy sensual pleasures and avoid pain and suffering at all costs, or (ii) to practice complete asceticism and renounce pleasure. Whether or not people lived to such extremes in practice will be examined in the second and third sections of this thesis, by looking at various depictions of yogis and their practices.

---

[20] Dermot Killingley, "Karma and rebirth in the Upaniṣads," in *The Upanisads*, ed. Signe Cohen (London: Routledge, 2017).
[21] Stuart Ray Sarbacker, *Tracing the Path of Yoga: The History and Philosophy of Indian Mind-Body Discipline*. (State University of New York Press, 2021), 31.
[22] Surendranath Dasgupta, *A History of Indian Philosophy* 1 (Great Britain: Cambridge University Press, 1922), 75.

As early as records show, the philosophical, scholarly, and religious milieu in pre-modern South Asia was primarily an oral tradition which featured formal debates.[23] Thus, many of the textual works we have now were originally oral and only written hundreds of years after the ideas emerged. Despite that, the texts tend to read as if they were debates with each other, though they did not always explicitly name other schools, texts, or authors, as just stating the ideas themselves tended to be enough citation for contemporary readers to understand the debate context. Due to this style of conversant scholarship, it is possible to draw connections between which schools had access to each other and roughly when that connection occurred. Inter-religious dialogues will be mentioned in relevant textual analysis throughout this thesis.

1.2 *Bhagavad Gītā* (BG) (400 BCE–200 CE)

First, we must examine the *Bhagavad Gītā*, one chapter of the much larger epic poem, the *Mahābhārata*, which likely had multiple authors over a vast period, possibly beginning as early as the first millennium BCE. The original date of the creation of the BG has been speculated to be in the second or third centuries BCE, but there is not any certainty as to the date the discourse took the form we know it as now, and this early date is unlikely.[24] However, it is possible to place this as the earliest text in this thesis because it does not reference any specific yoga schools or texts, uses different terminology than the later texts, and seems to be promoting these philosophies and practices as if for the first time. The intellectual landscape of India at the time was in quick development. As mentioned in the introduction, the orthodox schools of thought and belief of the *Vedas* and *Upaniṣads* were most dominant, but they were beginning to be

[23] O'Brien-Kop, *Rethinking 'Classical Yoga' and Buddhism*, 10.
[24] M. V. Nadkarni, *The Bhagavad-Gita for the Modern Reader: History, Interpretations and Philosophy*. (London: Routledge India, 2019), 17. Nadkarni provides a detailed analysis of the reasons other scholars have pushed for the date of this text, including comparing it to other traditions and intertextual studies.

challenged by alternative points of view. The BG, then, can be thought of as a response to these changing dialogues—as a way to make the orthodox wisdom make more sense and be more accessible to the average person (not just brahmins, for example).

The setting of the story is a battlefield in Kurukṣetra where Arjuna, the lead warrior of the Pāṇḍava family, is in conversation with his charioteer Kṛṣṇa, who is an incarnation of the Hindu deity Vishnu, and questions why he should fight. In his response, Kṛṣṇa details what the human condition is, how to follow our *dharma* (duty), and most importantly for our purpose, he introduces three ways to practice yoga with the goal of avoiding the "bonds of action."[25] Yoga, in the setting of the BG, is described as the means of putting philosophy into action for the purpose of deeply understanding the reality we live in and thus being able to disconnect from the habitual patterns that cause us harm. Simply put,

> *buddhiyukto jahātīha ubhe sukṛtaduṣkṛte*
> *tasmād yogāya yujyasva yogaḥ karmasu kauśalam* || 2.50 ||
>
> In this life, endowed with the intellect, one abandons both merits and evil actions. Thus, perform for the sake of yoga, for yoga is the skillfulness in every action.

The goal of practicing yoga is *jñānam* (wisdom) because with wisdom comes *śāntiḥ* (peace), which subsequently leads to *mokṣa* (liberation) from rebirth:

> *śraddhāvān labhate jñānaṃ tatparaḥ saṃyatendriyaḥ* |
> *jñānaṃ labdhvā parāṁ śāntim acireṇādhigacchati* || 4.39 ||
>
> That faithful one who is devoted and has controlled senses, attains knowledge. Having attained knowledge, he achieves supreme peace without delay.

According to the BG, rebirth is caused by improper actions which lead to consequences that must be played out, kind of like dominoes. If the domino falls in the wrong place, it causes a chain reaction that makes all the other dominos fall over all the way down the line. There are

---

[25] Patton, *The Bhagavad Gita*, 27.

infinite dominos in this philosophy and the only way to remove further dominos altogether is by engaging in one (or all) of the three paths of yoga described in the BG and detailed below. These paths are *karma* yoga, the yoga of action; *jñāna* yoga, the yoga of knowledge; and *bhakti* yoga, the yoga of devotion.

1.2.1 Karma Yoga

The first form of yoga described is that of karma, or action. Since the setting is a battle in which Arjuna is reluctant to participate, the first teaching is appropriately about how one should act. Kṛṣṇa says that if we act with the intent of particular outcomes, we will only cause our rebirth. Likewise, inaction is still a form of action, and one in which we are still attached to the results.

> *karmaṇy evādhikāras te mā phaleṣu kadācana* |
> *mā karmaphalahetur bhūr mā te saṅgo 'stv akarmaṇi* || 2.47 ||
>
> "Your authority is in action alone, and never in its fruits; motive should never be in the fruits of action, nor should you cling to inaction."[26]

Rather, we should act as our dharma requires without clinging to the results of our actions:

> *yogasthaḥ kuru karmāṇi saṅgaṃ tyaktvā dhanañjaya* |
> *siddhyasiddhyoḥ samo bhūtvā samatvaṃ yoga ucyate* || 2.48 ||
>
> "Abiding in yoga, engage in actions! Let go of clinging, and let fulfilment and frustration be the same; for it is said yoga is equanimity."[27]

---

[26] Patton, *The Bhagavad Gita*, 29.
[27] Patton, *The Bhagavad Gita*, 29. Note that *yogasthaḥ* (established in yoga) and *dhanañjaya* (O Arjuna) are missing from Patton's translation.

1.2.2 Jñāna Yoga

While karma yoga is the path of worldly action, the path that is interested in the mind is that of insight or wisdom (jñāna) of the self; to know the distinction between the doer of action and the action itself. Patton's translation notes that this is the practice of Sāṃkhya, while karma yoga is the practice of yoga:

> *yat sāṅkhyaiḥ prāpyate sthānaṃ tadyogair api gamyate* |
> *ekaṃ sāṅkhyaṃ ca yogaṃ ca yaḥ paśyati sa paśyati* || 5.5 ||
>
> "Those who practice *yoga* reach the place attained by those who practice *sāṃkhya*. The one who sees that *sāṃkhya* and yoga are one sees rightly."[28]

It would seem that karma yoga and jñāna yoga go hand in hand. One cannot participate in proper action without knowing what proper action is; thus, knowledge is required to perform proper action. It is also important to note that in this earliest description of yoga as a formal practice, the philosophy of Sāṃkhya and the practice of yoga are intimately linked. As in the verse (BG 5.5) above, the practice of yoga is one means to understand the philosophy of Sāṃkhya. While yoga as a unique school of practice and belief is not prevalent at this time yet, the idea of yoga practice as a tool to understand philosophies is evident.

1.2.3 Bhakti Yoga

The best practice of yoga is that of devotion, *bhakti*:

> *śreyo hi jñānam abhyāsāj jñānād dhyānaṃ viśiṣyate* |
> *dhyānāt karmaphalatyāgas tyāgāc cāntir anantaram* || 12.12 ||
>
> "Wisdom (jñāna) is better than practice, and focused mind is better than wisdom. Letting go of the fruit of action is better than a focused mind. From letting go, peace soon comes."[29]

---

[28] Patton, *The Bhagavad Gita*, 62.
[29] Patton, *The Bhagavad Gita*, 142.

"Focused mind" here means a singular focus on Kṛṣṇa's divine form. As noted by Zaehner (1969), this verse is kind of odd in that it does not mention the word "bhakti" specifically, but it can be extrapolated based on the context that "focused mind" is meant to indicate a singular focus on God, namely Kṛṣṇa.[30] "Bhakti" comes from the root √*bhaj*, "divide" or "grant. In its *ātmanepada* grammatical form, it can also mean "receive" or "enjoy." It can also mean "attend to," as in how one might serve a king. Bhakti as a practice is all these things—dividing the sacrificial offerings, enjoying the divine, and attending to the divine.[31] In the BG, the bhakti practitioners have no desires for themselves and no attachment to their senses. They do not believe in an "I" that exists separately from Kṛṣṇa, and thus their actions are fruitless and they are wise. Bhakti as a tradition allows any individual to choose their own personal deity—that which they most identify with—and worship it as a form of the divine. Bhakti has taken many forms over the years, but in the BG, it is a form of yoga that, if practiced without attachment to oneself, will lead one to liberation.

1.2.4 BG Context

In the *Mahābhārata*, the text in which the BG is a chapter, there are descriptions of *āsanas* (postures) that are meant to prepare the body for *yogasādhana*, a type of extended meditation.[32] These are not the first descriptions of such practices, as there were similar descriptions in the Upaniṣads and other earlier texts, but the existence of the descriptions here,

---

[30] Robert Charles Zaehner. *The Bhagavad-Gītā: With a Commentary Based on the Original Sources*. (Oxford: Clarendon Press, 1969), 329.

[31] Richard H. Davis, "Introduction: A Brief History of Religions in India," in *Religions of India in Practice* (Berkeley: Princeton University Press, 1995), 29.

[32] For example, see Droṇa Parva 192.51 and Bhīṣma Parva 30.13-14, as per Trikhā, *Mahābhārat Meṃ Yogavidhyā*, 23.

where yoga as a distinct practice is taught by Kṛṣṇa, formalizes the postures as part of a forming school of practice in a new way. It is important to note that these were not the poses we consider as part of haṭha yoga, as in they are not a series of āsanas for the sake of physical exertion. Rather, these are postures that are meant to allow for more productive meditation by keeping the body at ease.

Additionally, magical powers such as flight, controlling another's body, and controlling the elements are present throughout the text and are considered "yogic powers."[33] The Sanskrit terms used for these powers includes "*bala* (power, strength), *aiśvarya* (lordship, sovereignty), *vibhūti* (power, manifestation of power), *vīrya* (might), *prabhāva* (force) and, not infrequently, *yoga*."[34] This theme continues in all yoga texts, though the later texts adopt the word *siddhi* (here meaning "accomplishment;" later it comes to mean "supernatural powers") in place of many of these terms.[35] An important note, as Malinar (2012) details, is that these magic powers are not reminiscent of some "archaic magical thinking" but rather are explained quite simply by the fact that success in yoga means you become unified with *prakṛti* (nature/matter), and it is prakṛti that manages the elements. So, these magic powers are not supernatural but are quite simply the ability to see past the supposed distinction between our bodies and the world around us and become one with brahman.[36]

We see that in this early stage of literature on yoga, yoga is not a set of beliefs or practices separate from the Upaniṣadic philosophy of the time, but rather a tool used within the already established religious context. It would thus be inaccurate to say that yoga existed as its

---

[33] Angelika Malinar, "Yoga Powers in the Mahābhārata," in *Yoga Powers: Extraordinary Capacities Attained Through Meditation and Concentration*, edited by Knut A. Jacobsen, 33-60 (Lieden and Boston: Brill, 2012), 33.
[34] Malinar, "Yoga Powers in the Mahābhārata," 33.
[35] Malinar, "Yoga Powers in the Mahābhārata," 33.
[36] Malinar, "Yoga Powers in the Mahābhārata," 34.

own school at this point in history. However, it is important to be aware that the idea of these practices as a moral framework and a guideline to how to live life is already in the cultural milieu. As we will see in the next few primary texts, these ideas become more distinct as they begin to be codified into their own unique philosophies and more defined practices.

1.3 *Vaiśeṣika Sūtra* (VS) (2nd century CE)

The author of the *Vaiśeṣika Sūtra* is a philosopher by the name Kaṇāda Kāśyapa, and later commentators and scholars may refer to either name (amongst others).[37] This is a foundational text of the Vaiśeṣika school of Hindu philosophy, including theories about epistemology, atomism, realism, and ontology. It was the first text to fully develop an atomistic approach to philosophy in that all things can be divided down to increasingly smaller parts. At the same time, Kaṇāda recognized that there must be something which cannot be further divided, and he claimed that was the ātman. Some of the contents are critiques of Sāṃkhya philosophy, which is why it is important to include here because yoga and Sāṃkhya are heavily linked. The VS also describes the nature of yoga and the goal of *mokṣa* (liberation). Likely, the VS was written after the BG, but still before yoga was codified as a distinct school of thought and practice.[38] This timeline is useful to help place the development of the philosophical ideas that influenced the emergence of the yoga schools.

This school of philosophy takes its name from *viśeṣa*, which means "special characteristic," because it developed a "system of ontological classification, wherein the objects of experience are reduced to their fundamental categories."[39] In other words, the VS details what

[37] Bimal Krishna Matilal, *Nyāya-Vaiśeṣika*, edited by Jan Gonda (Wiesbaden: Harrassowitz, 1977), 54.
[38] Matilal, *Nyāya-Vaiśeṣika*, 55.
[39] Mikel Burley, *Haṭha-Yoga: Its Context, Theory and Practice* (Delhi: Motilal Banarsidass Publishers, 2000), 48.

things are and how we know they are that way. This introduced an atomistic way of understanding the world. Our relation to those categories is determined by valid knowledge, of which VS posits five kinds: perception, inference, remembrance, intuitive knowledge, and—the reason it is included in this thesis—yogic perception.[40] This is considered one of the "extraordinary perceptions." This school accepts three kinds of extraordinary perception: *sāmānyalakṣaṇa* (specific characteristics), *jñānalakṣaṇa* (intuitive knowledge), and *yogaja* (produced by yoga).[41] It is the last of these, yogaja, that allows yogis to perceive "the viśeṣas and atoms." "Viśeṣas" here refers to the qualities which all things are composed of (*guṇas*), which are *tamas* (inactivity), *rajas* (activity), and *sattva* (purity).[42]

The discussion about yoga is introduced in section two of chapter five of the VS, which is concerned with action and motion. Yoga is referenced in relation to seemingly "odd movements" which elude obvious description, such as magnetic forces and heat rising. It is not particularly clear if this is meant to suggest the concept of the magical abilities of advanced yogis was present at this time,[43] or if this is just suggesting that the yogis are aware of these forces because they are more educated. As we saw in the BG, the concept of having magical powers was possible, but it was not necessarily restricted to yogis, nor to these specific "odd movements." The only time yoga is specifically defined in the VS is the following:

> *tadanārambha ātmasthe manasi śarīrasya duḥkhābhāvaḥ saṃyogaḥ* || 5.2.16 ||
>
> "Yoga is defined as the lack of pleasure and pain when the mind is in a state of complete inaction within the self."[44]

---

[40] Krishna Prakash Bahadur, *The Wisdom of Sānkhya* (New Delhi: Sterling Publishers Pvt Ltd., 1978), 15.
[41] Kumār, *Classical Vaiśeṣika in Indian Philosophy*, 33.
[42] Bahadur, *The Wisdom of Sānkhya*, 17.
[43] By the time of Patañjali's *Yoga Sutras*, it is recognized that advanced yoga practitioners have abilities such as flight, transmutation, and mind-reading. More detail about those abilities will be provided in the PYS section. The inclusion of "odd movements" here in relation to seemingly indescribable phenomena suggest there may have been an idea of magical abilities already, even though it is not explicit.
[44] Matilal, *Nyāya-Vaiśeṣika*, 58.

The idea of mokṣa is also discussed in this section alongside yoga and is described as the state in which the self is no longer connected to the body and will not be connected to a new body after death, through rebirth.[45] This is congruent with the descriptions in the Gītā, such as in (BG 7.29):

> *jarāmaraṇamokṣhāya mām āśritya yatanti ye |*
> *te brahma tad viduḥ kṛitsnam adhyātmaṃ karma cākhilam* || 7.29 ||
>
> "Those who move towards freedom (mokṣa) from aging and death, resorting to me, know this brahman completely; they know the highest self and the entirety of action."[46]

Moḳsa was an idea that permeated South Asian thought, and the VS adopted it to mean that the person who achieves mokṣa does not identify with the body anymore:

> *tadabhāve saṃyogābhāvo 'prādurbhāvaś ca mokṣaḥ* || 5.2.18 ||
>
> Liberation is the absence of reincarnation which is caused by the absence of union [between the physical body and the causal body].[47]

The other major idea that circulated was that of *karma*, most simply defined as "action," and it is that definition which the VS uses. The soul is separate and distinct from the physical world and brahman, in the VS, and it is affected by voluntary actions (karma) which bring rise to consequences.[48]

1.4 *Sāṃkhyakārikā* (SK) (3rd century CE)

The *Sāṃkhyakārikā* was written by Iśvarakṛṣṇa.[49] Similar to the Vaiśeṣika Sūtra, the *Sāṃkhyakārikā* is not a yoga treatise as such, but the philosophy expounded in this text works alongside the practice and belief system of yoga. While Sāṃkhya is claimed to be the oldest Indian philosophical system, it is unlikely that there was a single original school of thought from

45 Matilal, *Nyāya-Vaiśeṣika*, 58.
46 Patton, *The Bhagavad Gita*, 92.
47 Bracketed text is due to the *tadabhāve* referencing the verse prior, not included here.
48 Bahadur, *The Wisdom of Sānkhya*, 16.
49 Burley, *Haṭha-Yoga*, 42.

which all other systems grew.[50] Likely, the development of the Sāṃkhya system occurred over a period of hundreds of years and so what specific ideas the yogis encountered is not necessarily clear. This text was likely composed after the VS, but they are roughly contemporary, and the philosophies were certainly prevalent before these texts were written.

There are certain themes that remain consistent throughout the history of Sāṃkhya thought that we will examine here, such as the cause of the cosmos and detachment from sense-objects.[51] Overall, this text considers reason to be our tool for understanding the world and shares similarities with the VS. But it departs from the VS's view of distinction of categories and things, instead viewing everything as one whole.[52] One of the ideas in the SK that is echoed in later yoga texts is:

> *puruṣasya darśanārthaṃ kaivalyārthaṃ tathā pradhānasya* |
> *paṅgvandhavad ubhayor api saṃyogas tatkṛtaḥ sargaḥ* || 21 ||
>
> "(The union) of the Spirit (with the Nature) is for contemplation (of the Nature); (the union) of the Nature (with the Spirit) is for liberation. The union of both (i.e., the Spirit and the Nature) is like that of a lame man with a blind man. The creation is brought about by that (union)."[53]

The Sanskrit used for "liberation" in SK is *kaivalya*,[54] whereas the Vaiśeṣika Sūtra uses *mokṣa*. When looking at Maas's critical edition of the PYS, kaivalya is used many more times than mokṣa.[55] Despite the concept being relatively the same, the language indicates that indeed the PYS favoured the Sāṃkhya terminology over the Vaiśeṣika. Additionally, this philosophy of

[50] Mikel Burley, *Classical Yoga and Sāṃkhya: An Indian Metaphysics of Experience*. (Oxon: Routledge, 2007), 13.
[51] Malinar, "Yoga Powers in the Mahābhārata," 41.
[52] Bahadur, *The Wisdom of Sānkhya*, 17.
[53] Sharma, *The Sāṃkhya-Kārikā*, Part III, 33.
[54] Sharma, *The Sāṃkhya-Kārikā*, Part II, 23.
[55] For instance, Maas (2006) compiled the colophon about the fourth pāda (chapter) in such a way to suggest it is about "kaivalya" rather than "mokṣa." Indeed, none of the alternative readings have "mokṣa": *iti pātañjale yogaśāstre sāṃkhyapravacane kaivalyapādaś caturthaḥ* || (pg xviii).

union is present in yogic thought as well, as we saw as early as the BG and will see as late as the *Haṭhayogapradīpikā*.

Indeed, the idea of *puruṣa* (spirit/consciousness) and prakṛti is detailed in Sāṃkhya philosophy as two distinct aspects and is most interested in defining the human condition in relation to these two aspects. Understandably, then, the SK deals heavily with theories of mind that later yoga texts pull from. For instance, *kārikā* 23 discusses the intellect. One part of intellect that is included in its sāttvika form is virtue. The text does not go into detail about what virtue means, or any other kinds of behaviour, however, the *Gauḍapāda-bhāṣya* commentary (c. sixth century CE) mentions that virtue includes "mercy, charity, the (five) *yamas* (restraints), and the (five) *niyamas* (obligations)... [which] are described in the treatise of Patañjali."[56] In other words, the SK does not mention those virtues specifically, but rather the commentator reads them into the philosophy. The commentator lived around 500 CE which is well after the original text was likely composed, and certainly after the PYS was composed.[57] Most likely, then, the *Sāṃkhyakārikā* is the earliest text, then the PYS, then *Gauḍapāda-bhāṣya*, so the commentator is reading the PYS into the *Sāṃkhyakārikā* as if the content of the PYS was what was intended all along, even though the PYS and *Sāṃkhyakārikā* were likely written at least a hundred years apart. This may suggest that the SK was unaware of yoga philosophy, but more intertextual study will need to be completed to determine that with any certainty.

In the SK, and Sāṃkhya philosophy as a whole, the goal is to understand the cause of existence in order to become liberated from the suffering that exists due to our misunderstanding:

[56] Sharma, *The Sāṃkhya-Kārikā*, Part III, 36. The commentary cites PYS II, 30 for yamas and 32 for niyamas.
[57] Sharma, *The Sāṃkhya-Kārikā*, 50.

duḥkhatrayābhighātāj jijñāsā tadabhighātake hetau |
dṛṣṭe sā 'pārthā cen naikāntātyantato 'bhāvāt || 1 ||

There is a desire to know the method to remove the pain caused by the three kinds of suffering. If [the desire to know is] said to be useless because obvious methods exist, this is not so, because those methods are not certain or permanent.

dṛṣṭavad ānuśravikaḥ sa hy aviśuddhikṣayātiśayayuktaḥ |
tadviparītaḥ śreyān vyaktāvyaktajñavijñānāt || 2 ||

The known methods are linked to impurity, decay, and excess. Indeed, the preferable means are from knowing the manifest, the unmanifest, and the knower.

The three kinds of suffering in Sāṃkhya philosophy are *ādhyātmika* (spiritual), *ādhidaivika* (supernatural), and *ādhibhautika* (physical).[58] Ādhyātmika suffering refers to the ailments of body and mind, such as sickness and anxiety. Ādhidaivika refers to suffering caused by uncontrollable external sources, such as environmental disasters. Ādhibhautika refers to the suffering caused by relatively controllable external sources, such as wild animals and thieves. The "known methods" listed in SK verse two as insufficient for overcoming suffering are primarily Vedic rituals—especially animal sacrifice. It states that the only way to overcome suffering is by knowing the distinction and relationship between the *vyakta* (the manifest; material world), prakṛti (the unmanifest, *avyakta*), and puruṣa (the knower, *jña*). While the VS thought that someone only needed to *understand* these concepts to become liberated, the SK wants people to practically experience them. The specific practices the SK mentions are as follows:

ādhyātmikāś catasraḥ prakṛtyupādānakālabhāgyākhyāḥ |
bāhyā viṣayoparamāt pañca nava tuṣṭayo 'bhimatāḥ || 50 ||

Nine appropriate types of spiritual satisfaction are known: five are external to the cessation of the sense objects, four are named prakṛti, clinging, time, and fortune.

[58] Kapila Vatsyayan, editor, *Kalātattvakośa: A Lexicon of Fundamental Concepts of the Indian Arts* 4 (Delhi: Indira Gandhi National Centre for the Arts and Motilal Banarsidass Publishers, 1988), 230.

ūhaḥ śabdo 'dhyayanaṃ duḥkhavighātās trayaḥ suhṛtprāptiḥ |
dānaṃ ca siddhayo 'ṣṭau siddheḥ pūrvo 'ṅkuśas trividhaḥ || 51 ||

Inference, instructions, studying, removal of three types of suffering, attainment of friends, and generosity are the eight means of accomplishment. The earlier ones are three kinds of restraints (of siddhi, supernatural powers).

The practical experience listed here pertains to becoming completely detached from sense-objects, often achieved through various kinds of meditation and asceticism. While detachment remains an idea in later yoga texts, the yogis of later texts more importantly believe they need to *master* their senses in order to achieve liberation, which is a slight but important distinction which shows that the SK and yoga philosophies are not necessarily completely overlapped.[59] A deeper analysis of the distinctions is outside the scope of this thesis.[60]

1.5 *Pātañjala Yogaśāstra* (PYS) (4th century CE)

Pātañjali's *Yogasūtras* is considered the original treatise on yoga practices, or at least the earliest that institutionalizes the practice as one distinct from other spiritual, religious, and physical-practice paths. The dating of PYS is highly contested. [61] A grammatical text written around the 2nd century BCE, called the *Mahābhāṣya*, is also attributed to someone by the name Patañjali, but scholars like Deshpande (2022) debate whether they are the same person or not.[62] Other schools of thought that were also ascetic traditions—the Śramaṇa traditions mentioned earlier—were also grappling with how to cease the churning of thoughts that so distract us

[59] Malinar, "Yoga Powers in the Mahābhārata," 41-2.
[60] Burley (2007) has done extensive analysis.
[61] For a comprehensive overview of the arguments, see Philip A. Maas, "A Concise Historiography of Classical Yoga Philosophy," 2013.
[62] Madhav Deshpande, "Language and Testimony in Classical Indian Philosophy", *The Stanford Encyclopedia of Philosophy*. Edited by Edward N. Zalta & Uri Nodelman (Fall 2022 Edition) https://plato.stanford.edu/archives/fall2022/entries/language-india/

humans from our true forms. These śramaṇa movements began around 500 BCE and were in dialogue among themselves and with each other well into the twelfth century CE; various scholars have tried to place PYS in time with the emergence of these conversations, but evidence is lacking; [63] the primary argument seems to be the topics covered, which, while the topics were part of the intellectual life of the first millennium BCE, this does not mean that the text that is discussing these topics must necessarily originate in that time period, as any scholastic piece, such as this thesis, for example, will be discussing older ideas and concepts.

More convincing is Maas's argument that the first known commentary on PYS, attributed to Vyāsa, was actually one and the same text, called *Pātañjala Yogaśāstra*, composed between 325 and 425 CE.[64] Maas's argument is based on intertextual analysis, in that authors contemporary to the PYS refer to it as a whole. Most likely, the ideas presented in the PYS were actively taught and practiced before the text was written, and the text acted more as an edited compendium with a commentary than a new text of its own. While we have philosophical texts that mention yoga before the PYS, we do not really have texts that speak of it in a substantial way as its own device. Perhaps further research can be done with regards to the gap between the BG and PYS, if indeed there were a few hundred years between the two.

Regardless of the date or the authorship, the most important part of PYS for the sake of this thesis is the practices and desires it espouses. PYS is separated into four *pāda*-s, or chapters, and contains one-hundred-and-ninety-five aphorisms. The first, called the *Samādhipāda*, is concerned with the primary questions of what yoga is, who can practice it, why someone would practice it, and how to practice it. The second chapter, called the *Sādhanāpāda*, is concerned with the practices themselves, such as the eight limbs, morals, breath work, and meditation.

---

[63] Sarbacker, *Tracing the Path of Yoga*, 127.

[64] Maas, "A Concise Historiography of Classical Yoga Philosophy," 66.

Chapter three, the *Vibhūtipāda* is concerned with the powers achieved by advanced yogis. The final chapter, the *Kaivalyapāda*, is concerned with the final goal of yoga practice, which is generally called samādhi, but as we saw earlier, also called kaivalya. In the case of PYS, samādhi means a type of deep meditation wherein the practitioner overcomes the physical limitations and exists as pure consciousness.

One of the main questions about the PYS we are concerned with is why it was written. The author was interested in compiling a set of practices and philosophies that appear to have been active in disaggregated ways for at least a few hundred years. The purpose of compiling them would have been to homogenize the practices into a formalized system. From the first line, it is clear the author deems there to be a conceptual gap in the available teachings (or perhaps no teachings available *en masse*, as we currently have no evidence for an established text before PYS) that will help people achieve union of their individual self with the universal self, and this text is meant to fill that gap. This is obvious from the first verse:

atha yogānuśāsanam || 1.1 ||

Now begins the instructions regarding yoga (union).[65]

The verse could have a few meanings. It could be that it is just beginning the text by saying "Now begins," or it could be that the author is hinting that they are starting something new in the trajectory of philosophical thought over time. Though an examination of the commentaries for this purpose is outside the scope of this thesis, it would be useful in future research. Regardless, the author does not keep us waiting. Naturally, the reader is thinking, "what

[65] This and all further Sanskrit of the PYS retrieved from Philip Maas, *Samādhipāda. Das erste Kapitel des Pātañjalayogaśāstra zum ersten Mal kritisch ediert. (Samādhipāda. The First Chapter of the Pātañjalayogaśāstra for the First Time Critically Edited).* (Aachen: Shaker, Studia Indologica Universitatis Halensis, Geisteskultur Indiens. Texte und Studien 9), 2006.

is this yoga you speak of?" Thankfully, the second verse tells us specifically what Patañjali's definition of yoga is:

> *yogaś cittavṛttinirodhaḥ* || 1.2 ||
>
> Yoga (union) is the cessation of the turnings of the mind.

The third verse tells us what the goal is, according to Patañjali:

> *tadā draṣṭuḥ svarūpe 'vasthānam* || 1.3 ||
>
> Then, the seer abides in its own form.

The rest of the sūtras explain how one achieves the cessation of the churning thoughts and what the outcomes of that practice are.

1.5.1 Teachings of PYS

The Yogasūtras lay out foundational practices of yoga, which include *yama* (moral principles), *niyama* (observances), *āsana* (posture), *prāṇāyāma* (breath control), *pratyāhāra* (withdrawal of the senses), *dhāraṇa* (concentration), *dhyāna* (meditation), and *samādhi* (pure contemplation). PYS touts that by practicing these teachings, one can be liberated from the material world and exist only as their puruṣa in true freedom.[66] This would give them supernatural powers because they would no longer be limited by the boundaries of possibility in the physical world. Why do we want to overcome the physical world? Because it is only in the physical world that suffering exists. It is important to note that Patañjali does recognize that physical reality has its own inherent existence, i.e., that objects are real. They are not just illusions, despite an accomplished yogi having the ability to modify them at will. It is these

[66] See, for instance, PYS 1.16 and 3.36 for descriptions of puruṣa.

special abilities that distinguishes many schools of yoga from the primarily physical practices we tend to associate with yoga today.

The āsanas described in the PYS have a contested history. While the commentary names thirteen postures, it may be that they were added by later glosses rather than Patañjali himself. Āsana itself is simply described as:

> *sthirasukham āsanam* || 2.46 ||
> *prayatnaśaithilyānantasamāpattibhyām* || 2.47 ||
>
> Posture (āsana) means to have motionlessness and good form.
> By relaxation of effort and meditation on the boundless[67] (āsanas are achieved).

And these are expanded upon in the commentary on PYS 2.47:[68]

> Either a posture is achieved because effort stops, whereby trembling of the body does not happen, or the mind, having merged meditatively into infinity, brings about the posture.[69]

So, the postures are not meant to be forced, nor are they practiced for the sake of the postures themselves. Specific postures were not even named in the original sutras, but only in the later commentaries (unless of course Maas is correct that the first commentary was the author himself). Rather, the postures are meant to be achieved either for the sake of extended periods of meditation and breathwork, or because of withdrawal of the senses, concentration, meditation, or pure contemplation. Namely, these periods of meditation need to be uninterrupted by the physical environment (heat, cold, etc.) or by the need for food and water.[70]

---

[67] It is important to note that samāpatti is actually a form of Buddhist meditation wherein there are eight samāpatti-s. As examined in the "Buddhist Connection" and "Amṛtasiddhi" sections below, this may be another instance where PYS is inspired by Buddhism, or vice versa. (See Robert E. Buswell Jr. and Donald S. Lopez Jr. "*Samāpatti,*" *The Princeton Dictionary of Buddhism* (New Jersey: Princeton University Press, 2013), 746.)

[68] Maas (2013) notes that the *Yogaśāstra* commentary on the PYS is likely Patañjali's own. If Patañjali did describe the poses in the commentary, it changes the tone of the PYS and may not have been added by later commentators.

[69] Philipp A. Maas, "'Sthirasukham Āsanam': Posture and Performance in Classical Yoga and Beyond," *Yoga in Transformation*, edited by Karl Baier, Philipp A. Maas, and Karin Preisendanz. (Göttingen: Veröffentlichungen der Vienna University Press, 2018), 57.

[70] Maas, "'Sthirasukham Āsanam'," 86.

1.5.2 Sāṃkhya Connection

We saw instruction for meditation in the *Sāṃkhyakārikā* for very similar methods, particularly withdrawal of the senses. The SK arose from the dualistic school of philosophy that was prevalent at the time of Patañjali called Sāṃkhya. This school believed in two aspects of existence: puruṣa (spirit/consciousness) and prakṛti. Material nature in Sāṃkhya includes (i) the five elements of earth, air, fire, water, and space, and (ii) the "subtle sphere." It has traditionally been argued that Patañjali built his practice of yoga on the philosophical teachings in Sāṃkhya. However, some scholars have suggested that yoga is ontologically distinct from Sāṃkhya, more in line with Buddhist thought, which I will examine below.[71] Larson (1989) brings to light the fact that Sāṃkhya teachings were in a state of flux when the PYS was being written, so it is uncertain which sources the author had access to. Thus, while the PYS aligned itself with Sāṃkhya, it may not have been with the SK specifically.[72] It is generally believed that the two schools of thought go hand in hand, even as early as we saw in the BG, but it is important to note some discrepancies. While a comprehensive list of discrepancies between the SK and PYS is outside the breadth of this thesis, we can pinpoint one important distinction, which is the language for mind. The SK uses the Sanskrit term *mahat* to indicate the "great source of

[71] It is unfortunately beyond the scope of this thesis to go into the details of comparing Yogic and Buddhist thought, but a good starting point for interest is Koichi Yamashita, *Pātañjala Yoga Philosophy with Reference to Buddhism*, (Calcutta: Firma KLM, 1994). More recently, Karen O'Brien-Kop's *Rethinking 'Classical Yoga' and Buddhism: Meditation, Metaphors and Materiality*. London: Bloomsbury Academic, 2022.

[72] Gerald James Larson, "An Old Problem Revisited, the Relation between Sāṃkhya, Yoga, and Buddhism," *Studien zur Indologie und Iranistik* 15, 1989, 129–46.

ahaṃkāra, 'self-consciousness,' and *manas*, 'the mind'."[73] In contrast, yoga uses *citta*, which is more like intelligence itself rather than some animating factor.[74]

1.5.3 Buddhist Connection

Buddhism also uses *citta* rather than *mahat.* O'Brien-Kop does detailed work showing that not only is the language of the PYS adopted from Buddhism, the ideas seem to often be in direct alignment.[75] Both Patañjali and the Buddha share an agreement on what *citta* (mind) is and does. However, the divergence seems to arrive with how it functions. Since the Nikāyas are a-dualist in that they do not recognize a spirit or non-material aspect at all, let alone one that needs to be distinguished from the material or non-spiritual world, they will fundamentally disagree with PYS which believes in the non-material spirit. Despite this fundamental difference, their practices are almost exactly aligned. They share the same morals, meditation techniques, reasons for practicing, and end goals. It almost seems as if Patañjali was trying to make Buddhism "fit" for a Brahmanical audience.

Indeed, śramaṇa movements grew in response to the well-developed Vedic and Brahmanical schools of thought and practice in northwestern India. These orthodox schools were attached to materiality through rituals, *varṇas* (castes), and *āśramas* (the four stages of life), which are *brahmacarya* (student), *gṛhastha* (householder), *vāṇaprastha* (forest-dweller), and *sannyāsa* (renunciant).[76] Which stage a person is in depends on both their age and their

---

[73] "mahat," *Monier-Williams Sanskrit-English Dictionary*, 1899, retrieved online April 30, 2023: https://www.sanskrit-lexicon.uni-koeln.de/scans/MWScan/2020/web/webtc/indexcaller.php
[74] "citta," *Monier-Williams Sanskrit-English Dictionary*, 1899, retrieved online April 30, 2023: https://www.sanskrit-lexicon.uni-koeln.de/scans/MWScan/2020/web/webtc/indexcaller.php
[75] O'Brien-Kop, *Rethinking 'Classical Yoga' and Buddhism.*
[76] Patrick Olivelle, *The Asrama System: The History and Hermeneutics of a Religious Institution* (London: Oxford University Press, 1993), 9-10.

circumstances, and the stage determines what their *dharma* (duty) is. Ascetics operated outside of this framework, though their beliefs did not necessarily diverge as much as their practices did. Like the Vedic and Brahmanical schools, Patañjali believed in duality, that there is an eternal, continuous soul that is separate from physical reality. Unlike the Upaniṣadic schools which structure the relationship between the soul and matter as (i) brahman, (ii) ātman, and (iii) prakṛti, PYS does not speak of the ātman/brahman duality and instead renames this "ultimate consciousness," puruṣa (PYS 1.16).[77] Of course, Buddhism denies the idea of an individual, permanent soul. So, it is almost as if PYS conflates the two extremes to make it more appealing to a wider audience.

While the philosophies are obviously in conversation, the language itself is also borrowed. The PYS was composed originally in Sanskrit, as far as we know, but some of the terminology it uses is either non-Pāṇinian Sanskrit or not Sanskrit at all. For instance, Renou (1940) points out the word *muditā* (sympathetic joy) as not well-formed Sanskrit due to its feminine verbal noun form which is not usually seen in Classical Sanskrit. However, Edgerton (1953) and Wujastyk (2018) claim it is a perfectly fine form found in "Buddhist Hybrid Sanskrit," additionally suggesting PYS is influenced by Buddhism.[78] Wujastyk goes on to provide explanations for three other verses in PYS that use explicitly Buddhist terminology in a way that assumes the audience would not need further explanation of the terms since the audience would have sufficient understanding of Buddhist ideas. One such example was the use

---

[77] *tatparaṃ puruṣakhyāter guṇavaitṛṣṇyaṃ.*

[78] Louis Renou, "On the Identity of the Two Patañjalis," in *Louis de La Vallée Poussin Memorial Volume,* edited by N.N. Law, 368–373 (Calcutta: J. C. Sarkhel, 1940); Franklin Edgerton, *Buddhist Hybrid Sanskrit Grammar and Dictionary.* Vol. 2. *Dictionary.* William Dwight Whitney Linguistic Series. (New Haven: Yale University Press, 1953); Dominik Wujastyk, "Some Problematic Yoga Sūtra-s and Their Buddhist Background," in *Yoga in Transformation*, edited by Karl Baier, Philipp A. Maas, and Karin Preisendanz. (Göttingen: Veröffentlichungen der Vienna University Press, 2018).

of the term *dharmamegha* in Kaivalyapāda 29, which is a term only explicitly mentioned in the Mahāyāna Buddhist text *Daśabhūmikasūtra*, and indicates a particular kind of samādhi:[79]

> *prasaṅkhyāne 'py akusīdasya sarvathāvivekakhyāter dharmameghaḥ samādhiḥ* || 4.29 ||
>
> "He who has no investment even in contemplation, who has the realization of discrimination in every respect, obtains *dharmamegha samādhi*."[80]

This is not to say necessarily that Patañjali himself was Buddhist, but to hark back to the fact that debate was a main mode of scholarship, his use of Buddhist terminology and ideas is proof that he was at least in conversation with the Buddhists of the time. The conversation between yoga and Buddhism continues well through to the present day, and it is through Buddhism that tantric practices are eventually codified into haṭha yoga, as I will show in the analysis of the *Amṛtasiddhi* below.

1.6 *Amṛtasiddhi* (AS) (11th century CE)

As we have seen, yoga was originally a means to achieve liberation and was composed of various stages. While āsanas were included, they were limited and only for the purpose of preparing the body for extended periods of meditation. Yoga in PYS and contemporary texts were friendly to Upaniṣadic philosophies, while other Śramaṇa schools detracted from the mainstream Brahmanical system to forge new, opposing belief systems. Despite the differing beliefs, the practices were relatively similar. Ascetics operated within each of the traditions. However, some practices were more extreme or confined to a particular school of thought. Around the eleventh century, certain schools of Buddhism were infused with tantric practices

[79] See O'Brien-Kop, *Rethinking Classical Yoga and Buddhism*, 103 for an extensive analysis of the term.
[80] Wujastyk, "Some Problematic Yoga Sūtra-s and Their Buddhist Background," 35-6.

that were like Śaivite practices, and while they were similar, the Vajrayāna Buddhists codified some of the practices into treatises before Śaivism did. The earliest such Buddhist text is the AS and it appears to be where the more tantric physical practices of haṭha yoga were pulled from.[81] That is not to say that Śaivites did not practice these things as well, there just is not textual evidence of it being codified as it was in the AS. The AS was written in both Tibetan and Sanskrit and states the author as Mādhavacandra. Though we do not have any historical context as to who that is, Mallinson has argued that it was likely composed in the Deccan region of India.

Around the same time of the composition of the AS, Tibetan Buddhists were teaching "physically demanding preparatory exercises and prescribed postures… that push physiology – and thereby consciousness – beyond habitual limits," including sequential movements reminiscent of the yoga sequences used in modern-day haṭha yoga.[82] The term "haṭha-yoga" itself first appears in an eighth century Buddhist tantric text, the *Guhyasamājatantra*, as a "forceful" means of attaining visions, awakening, and insight.[83]

One of the things the AS does that earlier tantric texts do not do is codify the yogic body as a triad of sun, moon and fire.[84] It also connects the idea of *bindu* (sexual fluids—both male and female) to this "yoga body," expanding the concept of body to be connected with the mind and breath.[85] Mallinson (2020) gives a comprehensive review of other things it does differently, such as various postures and breath control.[86] Additionally, the AS also does not mention *cakras* (energetic wheels) or *kuṇḍalinī* (the energetic coil at the base of the spine), themes consistent in

---

[81] Mallinson, *The Amṛtasiddhi*, 410.
[82] Ian A. Baker, "Tibetan Yoga: Somatic Practice in Vajrayāna Buddhism and Dzogchen," in *Yoga in Transformation*, edited by Karl Baier, Philipp A. Maas, and Karin Preisendanz (Göttingen: Veröffentlichungen der Vienna University Press, 2018), 338.
[83] Baker, "Tibetan Yoga," 339.
[84] Mallinson, *The Amṛtasiddhi*, 413-414.
[85] Mallinson, *The Amṛtasiddhi*, 414.
[86] James Mallinson, "The Amṛtasiddhi: Haṭhayoga's Tantric Buddhist Source Text," in *Śaivism and the Tantric Traditions: Essays in Honour of Alexis G.J.S. Sanderson*. Edited by Peter C. Bisschop. Brill Online, 2020

both earlier and later tantric texts.[87] While previous yoga texts considered the body to be an obstacle to yoga practice, the AS considers the body as a tool to assist in yoga practice due to the manipulation of the elements. This is a drastic shift that impacts yoga practices from then on.

1.7 *Yogavāsiṣṭha* (YV) (10th to 12th century CE)

The author of the YV is unknown, which makes dating the text particularly difficult. However, it is a pan-Indian rendering of the *Mokṣopāya*, a text composed prior to the tenth century CE.[88] Various versions of the text exist, some with as little as six-thousand verses and some up to thirty-two-thousand verses.[89] It is posited that it likely began in a short version, the original of which is now lost to us, and grew over time—possibly over centuries.[90] One such version is known as the *Laghu-Yogavāsiṣṭha* and *Mokṣopāya*. The YV is structured as a set of stories told to Rāma, the primary character of the Rāmayana, used as a mode to teach the underlying philosophy. Rāma, disappointed with the fact that human existence is suffering, approaches an ancient sage named Vasiṣṭha to ask how to become liberated from this cycle of dying and being reborn. Throughout the book, Rāma is taught the philosophies and practice of yoga until finally at the end he has attained enlightenment.

The ultimate goal of yoga in the YV is to realize there is "no division in space," in other words, prakṛti and puruṣa are not separate, and there is no self separate from brahman.[91] In fact, the external world is considered an illusion:

---

[87] Baker, "Tibetan Yoga," 343.

[88] Walter Slaje, "Liberation from Intentionality and Involvement: On the Concept of '*Jīvanmukti*' According to the *Mokṣopāya*," *Journal of Indian Philosophy* 28, no. 2 (April 2000), 171-194.

[89] Venkatesananda, *The Concise Yoga Vāsiṣṭha*, ix.

[90] Venkatesananda, *The Concise Yoga Vāsiṣṭha*, x.

[91] Venkatesananda, *Vasiṣṭha's Yoga*, 195.

yataḥ kutaścid ucchrāyaṃ gandharvapuravanmanaḥ |
bhrāntimātraṃ tanotīdaṃ jagadākhyaṃ svajṛmbhaṇam || 3.84.30 ||

"Whatever is in the mind is like a city in the clouds.
The emergence of this world is no more than thoughts manifesting themselves."[92]

The YV is nondualist, which is the opposite of PYS's stark dualism wherein prakṛti is separate from puruṣa, and puruṣa is part of brahman. According to this text, realizing nonduality allows a yogi to choose their own death; by practicing "the yoga of concentration and meditation [they will] depart [die] at their sweet will and pleasure."[93]

On a basic level, according to the YV, "Yoga is getting rid of the poison of desire."[94] The practices also remove fear and other afflictions of mind.[95] Additionally, the practice of yoga leads to the attainment of what might be considered magical powers, which is a theme we saw all the way back in the *Mahābhārata*. Something new in this text is that we see (and hear from) women who are successful practitioners of yoga, though whether or not it is a true distinction between genders is questionable as it is a nondualist text. One such example is when a formless woman describes how she became a yogi: "Because my husband had no interest in me, I developed dispassion. The mental conditioning became weak and I practiced yoga which conferred on me control over space, so that I can move in space."[96] In other words, practicing yoga gave this woman the ability to fly, which is an ability commonly mentioned throughout the history of yoga.

What is the practice of yoga exactly, as dictated in this text? It is meditation, contemplation, and realization; self-knowledge. It mentions āsanas, though it does not describe

---

[92] Venkatesananda, *The Concise Yoga Vāsiṣṭha*, xiii.
[93] Venkatesananda, *Vasiṣṭha's Yoga*, 79.
[94] Venkatesananda, *Vasiṣṭha's Yoga*, 521.
[95] Venkatesananda, *Vasiṣṭha's Yoga*, 218.
[96] Venkatesananda, *Vasiṣṭha's Yoga*, 551.

which postures specifically are to be practiced since they are secret and should be taught by the guru.[97] This text only names the lotus posture, which is a seated position typically used for meditation, *prāṇāyāma* (breathwork), recitation of *mantras*, worship of images, and other visualization practices.[98] It also states to practice a pure diet, right conduct, and renunciation.[99]

The Yogavāsiṣtha specifically states this is all to be practiced "without the violence involved in Haṭha Yoga, for Haṭha Yoga gives rise to pain."[100] While the YV disagrees with haṭha yoga, the text specifically mentions Sāṃkhya philosophy, namely that the two philosophies agree on what puruṣa is. They agree that puruṣa is the same as brahman, pure consciousness, but Sāṃkhya is dual and believes something exists outside of the mind, i.e., the material world, while the YV is nondualist so thinks there is no distinction between mind and matter.[101]

1.8 *Haṭhapogapradīpikā* (HYP) (15th century CE)

This text is one of the first comprehensive treatises on haṭha yoga and it attributes itself in particular to the Nāth lineage.[102] The author is Svātmārāma, also known as Yogīndra, but since much of the content is borrowed (sometimes explicitly, sometimes not) from other texts, it may be more appropriate to call Svātmārāma an editor or commentator.[103] The content discusses the proper place to practice yoga, ethics, postures, prāṇāyāma, *mudrā* (energetic and physical "locks"), meditation, and samādhi.

---

[97] Venkatesananda, *Vasiṣṭha's Yoga*, 320.
[98] Venkatesananda, *Vasiṣṭha's Yoga*, 324.
[99] Venkatesananda, *Vasiṣṭha's Yoga*, 427.
[100] Venkatesananda, *Vasiṣṭha's Yoga*, 275.
[101] Venkatesananda, *Vasiṣṭha's Yoga*, 313.
[102] Sarbacker, *Tracing the Path of Yoga*, 170.
[103] Burley, *Haṭha-Yoga: Its Context, Theory and Practice*, 6.

The HYP describes sixteen different āsanas that are meant to be practiced until there is no more physical pain so that the practitioner can be comfortable in extended periods of meditation, eventually achieving Rāja Yoga.[104] It does note that these are not the only postures, just the ones the author, Svātmārāma, finds most important. At HYP 4.3-4, Rāja yoga is described as synonymous with samādhi, as well as several other terms.[105]

The inclusion of Rāja yoga is important to note because before this text, Rāja and haṭha yoga were at odds with each other, each claiming to be the superior path. It is in this text that the two schools are brought together as something that can be achieved in tandem.[106] In fact, later in the HYP, it even says there can be "no success in rāja-yoga without haṭha, nor in haṭha without rāja-yoga."[107] (HYP 2.76) The HYP also states that *āstikya* (orthodoxy, typically the belief in God) and study of the Upaniṣads are prerequisites for becoming a yogi.[108] In a way, it seems as if HYP is doing the same thing as the PYS—bring a bunch of teachings together to make it more applicable to wider audiences.

Samādhi is later described as "oneness of the self and the ultra self"—in other words, union.[109] In order to achieve samādhi, there are many practices a person must undertake. Included are ten yamas (moral principles):

> *ahiṃsā satyam asteyaṃ brahmacaryaṃ kṣamā dhṛtiḥ* |
> *dayārjavaṃ mitāhāraḥ śaucaṃ caiva yamā daśa* || 1.17 ||[110]
>
> Nonviolence, truthfulness, non-stealing, celibacy, forgiveness, patience, compassion, honesty, modest diet, and cleanliness are the ten moral values.

---

[104] Svātmārāma. *The Haṭha Yoga Pradīpikā*, trans. Sinh, iv.
[105] Svātmārāma, *The Hatha Yoga Pradīpikā*, trans. Sinh, 47
[106] Jason Birch, "The Meaning of *haṭha* in Early Haṭhayoga," *Journal of the American Oriental Society* 131, no 4 (2011), 527.
[107] Burley, *Haṭha-Yoga: Its Context, Theory and Practise*, 104.
[108] Burley, *Haṭha-Yoga: Its Context, Theory and Practise*, 43n.5.
[109] Svātmārāma. *The Haṭha Yoga Pradīpikā*, 47: Tatsamaṃ ca dvayor aikyaṃ jīvātmaparamātmanoḥ, pranaṣṭasarvasaṇkalpaḥ samādhiḥ so 'abhidhīyate. (7)
[110] Svātmārāma. *The Haṭha Yoga Pradīpikā*, 3.

It also mentions ten niyamas (observances):

> *tapaḥ saṃtoṣa āstikyaṃ dānam īśvarapūjanam |*
> *siddhāṃtavākyaśravaṇaṃ hrī matī ca japo hutam |*
> *niyamā daśa saṃproktā yogaśāstraviśāradaiḥ* || 1.18 ||[111]
>
> Penance, satisfaction, piety, charity, worship of God, listening to scriptures, modesty, intellect, ritual offering, and chanting are the ten observances according to people learned in yoga texts.

This is double the amount of yamas and niyamas found in PYS.

The āsanas described are attributed to sages and yogis such as Vasiṣṭha and Matsyendra.[112] While it is not clear from the text itself specifically who these are referring to, likely Vasiṣṭha is the author of the thirteenth-century text *Vāsiṣṭha Saṃhitā* that is one of the first texts to describe non-seated āsanas.[113] The "Matsyendra" the text refers to is likely Matsyendranāth, the founder of the Nāth *sampradāya* (lineage). So again, we are finding the HYP refer to a variety of sources across multiple philosophies and religious practices. While this is considered a breakthrough treatise on haṭha yoga, this suggests that it might be more appropriate to call it an attempt at unifying various practices into one whole.

1.9 Conclusions: History of Yoga

This section examined seven primary texts that consider themselves to be part of the yoga corpus or are directly impacted by or cause ruptures in yoga philosophy. While many concepts and teachings are the same, some important ones diverge. The table below helps us map the ideas to make it clearer where the overlaps and divergences are.

---

[111] The Pancham Sinh translation of the HYP (1915) has the reading "tapo hutam" but the Adyar Library edition (1972) has "japo hutam" so I am taking the latter reading as it is more coherent.
[112] Svātmārāma, *The Haṭha Yoga Pradīpikā*, 4.
[113] James Mallinson and Mark Singleton, *Roots of Yoga* (London, UK: Penguin Books, 2017), 257-8.

Table 2. Comparison of key concepts

Teaching[114]	**BG**	**VS**	**PYS**	**SK**	**AS**	**YV**	**HYP**
Duality	Dual	Dual	Dual	Dual	Nondual	Nondual	Nondual
Goal	mokṣa	mokṣa	samādhi	mokṣa	Prabhodhāyām / samādhi	mokṣa	mokṣa & samādhi
Powers	✓	✓	✓	✕	✓	✓	✓
Moral principles (yama)	~	~ only dharma	5	~	✕	✓	10
non-violence	✕	-	✓	-	-	✓	✓
truthfulness	-	-	✓	-	-	✓	✓
non-stealing	-	-	✓	-	-	✓	✓
celibacy	-	-	✓	-	-	~	✓
generosity	-	-	✓	-	-	✓	✓
Observances (niyama)	✕	✕	5	✕	✕	✓	10
cleanliness	-	-	✓	-	-	✕	~
contentment	-	-	✓	-	-	✕	✓
asceticism	-	-	✓	-	-	✓	✓
sacred study	✓	-	✓	-	-	✕	✓
dedication to God	✓	-	✓	-	-	✕	✓
Posture (āsana)	seated	-	seated	-	✓	✓	✓
Breath control (prāṇāyāma)	~	-	✓	-	✓	✓	✓

[114] Legend: ✓ = present, ✕ = not present/explicitly against, ~ = partially present/not explicit, - = not applicable

Teaching	BG	VS	PYS	SK	AS	YV	HYP
Sense withdrawal (pratyāhāra)	~	-	✓	-	×	✓	✓
Concentration (dhārāṇa)	✓	-	✓	×	×	✓	✓
Meditation (dhyāna)	✓	-	✓	×	✓	✓	×
Pure contemplation (samādhi)	~	~	✓	✓	✓	✓	✓

This table makes it clear that, while there are significant changes in what yoga is defined as, what its goal is, and how to achieve that goal, there is still a thread that goes throughout, building on the foundations laid before. For instance, the introduction of tantric ideas brought with it many more physical practices that were not just intended for the sake of calming the body to focus the mind, but also for the sake of energetic manipulation of the body and elements. The moral teachings also expanded as the practice of yoga became increasingly more codified and separate from the other philosophical and religious schools.

While many people want to claim that the yoga we practice today is an evolution of some millennia-old teaching, it is not quite that clear. More accurately, various philosophies were speaking about similar topics in similar ways and so it appears to be a more unified whole than it really was. As we can see in the examples above, some texts are reading newer texts into older ones (such as the SK reading PYS into VS) and some do not even mention the older ones altogether (such as the AS and PYS). It seems like the history of yoga is more about ruptures or radical new ideas changing the scenery rather than a linear evolutionary path.

The connection between Buddhism and Yoga is being researched actively, and while I could only touch upon it in this thesis, it is an interesting development as it explains where haṭha yoga received many of its teachings (i.e., tantric Buddhist practices). While we consider debates to be taking place in the ancient courts, it appears that these authors were debating ideas across religious boundaries even if they did not necessarily have official debates in courts anymore.

Śāstrārtha (intellectual court debates) were an important factor in the development of ideas in ancient India.[115] The courts themselves were also fundamental to discourse in general, as much of the poetry and literature that was produced in (and about) the courts speak about the people and ideas that were present in them. We will see some examples of this courtly poetry in both of the following sections. During the establishment of various Islamic states in South Asia between the eighth and fourteenth centuries, this role of political courts as sites of intellectual inquiry continued, though in a different form. Thus, as we examine texts in the following sections that were sometimes explicitly, and sometimes assumed to be, produced by court commissions, we will see that the courts—and intellectual life in general—viewed yoga philosophy as something worthy of discussing (sometimes arguing against, other times arguing for). They also tended to find yogis as particularly curious people with strange and extreme practices. The opinions about yogis and yoga philosophy we see in many of the texts examined later in this thesis are not all positive—in fact, many of them are openly derogatory towards these groups. While we cannot presume to know the true motivations behind these depictions, it is telling that they were depicted at all. Each case is unique, and I will do my best to analyze the depictions not only in relation to each other but as their own contained units.

[115] Radhavallabh Tripathi, *Vāda in Theory and Practice: Studies in Debates, Dialogues and Discussions in Indian Intellectual Discourses* (India: D.K. Printworld, 2021).

Overall, this section gave us a sense of what yoga is, what the goals are, what a yogi actually practiced, and what sort of attributes each tradition holds high in importance. While we examine literary texts in the following two sections, we can use this conceptual backdrop to compare the depictions of yogis in those texts to what the yogis would consider themselves to be like, and hopefully develop a better understanding of how accurately they were viewed by non-practitioners, or perhaps how accurately practitioners practiced their trade.

2 Early Islamicate Engagements with Yoga

In order to understand how a group of people actually practiced yoga, it is important to not just look at their own descriptions, or descriptions from people who are sympathetic towards them, but also look at how they were described by people that had differing beliefs about how to achieve similar goals. As historians realized in the mid-twentieth century, using texts to learn about the civilization within which they were written is problematic as it is limited to the views of the people who were able to write those texts—often the literary elites.[116] In an attempt to get a wider perspective on who yogis were and what they believed and practiced, this section will examine texts written by Islamicate scholars and Sufis.

I have chosen to look at Islamicate descriptions of yoga beliefs and practices, and their depictions of yogis as individual people, because Sufism—a mystical division of Islam— and yoga have similar beliefs and practices, such as asceticism, though with enough difference that the conversation between them has proven to be at once coherent in its depth of understanding while also being critical of some specific practices and beliefs. I believe, and hope to prove, that this comparative study will shed more light on how yoga was practiced than if I were to just examine Sanskrit literature. For instance, the Islamicate writings I look at are dealing in some sense with "othering" the yogis, either by recognizing that yogis are a new phenomenon they want to understand or trying to show that the yogis are not as successful or useful as the Sufis. I will use this othering framework to help analyze the Sanskrit sources also.

At the same time, I believe that studying these texts may say more about the authors writing them than about their subjects, but that can be equally useful in contextualizing the yogic context, even if indirectly. It is important to acknowledge clearly that this way of studying a

---

[116] Richard Eaton, *Essays on Islam and Indian History* (Cambridge: Oxford University Press, 2000), 11-12.

group of people as if they were a homogenous whole writing about another homogenous whole is a vast generalization at best and certainly incomplete, but it is an important piece of the puzzle that I hope can be used in a larger study examining the various pieces of data about yogis. I make every attempt to examine each text in its own heterogeneous context as well as its part in the evolution of zeitgeists.

This section will examine four primary texts that will be analyzed in order of their dates: Al-Bīrūnī's *Kitāb Bātanjal* (KB) from the eleventh century; "Medieval Sufi Tales of Jogis" translated by Simon Digby, originally completed in the twelfth and thirteenth centuries; Ghawth Gwaliyari's *Bahr al-hayat* from the fifteenth century; and Rājgīrī's *Madhumālatī* from the sixteenth century. These texts all deal with practitioners of yoga or the philosophy and practices of yoga, and show that the Sufis who were translating and opining on them tended to think their own beliefs and practices were superior. Though he was not a Sufi himself, it is important to include Al-Bīrūnī's KB in this examination of depictions of yogis because he was the first Islamicate scholar to do two things: first, he spent significant time learning from pandits not initially in order to compile this translation but at first for the sake of learning itself, and second, he was one of the first to structure the study of religion in a comparative manner that clearly defined different groups of people under specific religious frameworks.[117] Throughout all these texts, the physical practices of yoga were depicted as they were originally described, but the benefits, outcomes, and philosophical and religious beliefs surrounding them were either depicted explicitly as untrue, bad for the person, ignored altogether, or replaced by what the Sufis thought was more relevant and true—namely their Islamic philosophy. In fact, the word "yoga" rarely appears in Islamicate literature, but instead seems to be commonly replaced by the

[117] Senin, "Understanding the 'other': the case of Al-Biruni (973-1048 AD)," 394.

Arabic-Persian term *riyāzat* (ascetic practice), showing that the Sufis and other Persian commentators did not see yogis as a religious group separate from their own but rather as people who practice asceticism much like themselves.[118] This is an important distinction because the way that "othering" happens changes over time. The earliest text here shows the beginning of the "othering" process as a way to actually engage fairly—as acknowledged by al-Bīrūni himself—with the yogic texts while acknowledging a distinction between the "heretic," i.e., non-Muslim, beliefs, and the translator's own beliefs. Before al-Bīrūni, "others" were seen as inferior, but as we progress through the texts in this section, we see that they end up being completely accepting of yoga practice if not belief. Regardless, the overall theme seems to be the Sufis grappling with the idea of how these people who practice similar things can have such wildly different beliefs about them, writ large, without much nuance about the different schools of belief.

2.1 Background

2.1.1 Literature Review

The interactions between Sufis and yogis have been effectively documented by a number of scholars. Carl Ernst focuses on the similarities between Sufis and yogis as well as how other communities perceived them. Aditya Behl and Wendy Doniger shows how Sufis engaged with the "Indian cultural landscape [by] using local terms, symbols, concepts, techniques and gods," and particularly through the literature.[119] Simon Digby focuses on the Nāth yogis's relations with Sufis and how political factors influenced the exchange of ideas between the two groups, while

[118] Carl W. Ernst, "A Fourteenth Century Persian Account of Breath Control and Meditation," in *Yoga in Practice* (Princeton University Press, 2011), 133.
[119] Aditya Behl and Wendy Doniger, *Love's Subtle Magic: An Indian Islamic Literary Tradition, 1379-1545* (Oxford University Press, 2012), 1.

providing examples such as travel diaries and tales. Richard Eaton turns outwards and examine the ways that Sufis and yogis shaped political power through new modes of intellectual inquiry and the Persian language. Mario Kozah examines the inter-cultural and inter-religious dynamics with a particular interest in how Islamic scholarship impacted "othering," i.e., people's views of each other. Christine Marrewa-Karwoski analyzes lost texts that shed light on how Nāth yogis saw their relationship to Sufis. Noémie Verdon and Philip Maas looked at how al-Biruni and his contemporary scholars shaped the narrative between Sufis and yogis. Shankar Nair focused on how Sufis and yogis spoke to each other and interacted with their shared political power structures, with more emphasis on similarities rather than differences. Daniela Bevilacqua focused on Nāth yogis, haṭha yoga, and their ascetic and mystical practices. William Chittick studied Sufi poetry in particular and how it spoke (or did not speak) to how Sufis practiced, what their context was, and what their beliefs about other groups were. Zaehner compared Hindu and Muslim mysticism writ large, without just focusing on Nāths and Sufis. Many other scholars have done more work, but this section will build primarily upon these works. All are referenced multiple times in the bibliography.

While those scholars focused on religious, political, or physical angles of analysis, what I am primarily interested in is the topic of yoga and yogis, and the process of how Sufis positioned themselves in relation to this group through their own writings. While it is true that Sufis arrived in India long after the development of yogic practice and beliefs, it is generally recognized in modern scholarship that we cannot accurately view religious expansion as a "flowing outward from some central point" but rather as how a society in the place and time of interest was undergoing change.[120]

[120] Eaton, *Essays on Islam and Indian History,* 46.

2.1.2 Historical Context

From the texts analyzed in this section, we can see that Sufis did not position themselves as "outsiders" in conflict with "locals." Recent scholarship, such as Eaton (2000) suggests that indeed Muslims over history (and particularly before European colonization) did not conceive of their identities as nation states, but rather the "global nature of *umma*," i.e. "the community of believers."[121] Thus, yogis were not initially positioned as something alien or other because of their "yoginess," so to speak, but as whether or not they would conform to and accept the Muslim societal structures and rulership. Since Sufis were often the harbingers of "Mughal imperial influence and the Persianized culture associated with it,"[122] it is reasonable to approach the writings in this section as indicative of how two cultures "creatively adapted" to each other.[123]

Keeping in view the long history of engagements between Islamicate and Sanskritic philosophical traditions that occurred under the Abbasid Caliphate as early as the eighth and ninth centuries, I will refrain from viewing early modern Sufi references to yoga as representative of an overarching original Muslim cultural encounter. Indeed, the Muslim caliphate in Baghdad assimilated knowledge from all over the contacted world, translating texts from Sanskrit, Greek, and many other languages, into Arabic.[124] As the Caliphate expanded in territory and contacted and assimilated other cultures, they inherited the Sasanians' policy toward

---

[121] Eaton, *Essays on Islam and Indian History,* 44.
[122] Eaton, *Essays on Islam and Indian History,* 37.
[123] "Creative adaptation" is a concept from John Smail that describes the acceptance of change by groups of people coming into contact with each other. Smail developed this idea about Southeast Asia, but Richard Eaton suggests this applies equally to the South Asian context and perhaps all Muslim communities. (John R.W. Smail, "On the Possibility of an Autonomous History of Modern Southeast Asia," *Journal of Southeast Asian History* 2, no. 2 (July 1961); Eaton, *Essays on Islam and Indian History,* 44).
[124] Eaton, *Essays on Islam and Indian History,* 28-9.

minorities in that the ruler "extended to the communities recognition, tolerance, and protection in return for political loyalty and taxes."[125] While this did not mean that all communities passively chose to follow the Muslim imperial rule, the Muslim courts themselves were not necessarily hostile towards other communities. With this in mind, I will examine each text in its own context regarding how it approaches the yogic community rather than as a specifically Muslim-centric text with some kind of imposing philosophy.

As Sufism was developing into a more codified religious practice, Muslims were traveling internationally as traders and Sufis tended to travel with them. Ports of trade were being established all across Eurasia that encouraged freer movement of both people and goods. The first maritime contact with South Asia by Arab merchants was in the eighth century, and with merchants often came other travelers—scholars, politicians, and religious missionaries.[126] Sufis, since they were ascetics and thus not attached to worldly goods such as houses and kingdoms, were extremely mobile. They tended to travel with merchants and were often the first contact of Islamic religion in new places.[127] Port cities, and soon in-land cities, were established or broadened by Muslims.

2.1.3 What is Sufism and How Does it Compare to Yoga?

Though each text and author are unique in their perspective and understanding, there are some generalizations about Sufis and yogis that can and should be made to help contextualize these texts. Sufis and yogis are similar in their asceticism and mysticism, but they differ in their conception of the final goal of their practice and how exactly to achieve that goal. On a broad,

---

[125] Eaton, *Essays on Islam and Indian History,* 24.
[126] Eaton, *Essays on Islam and Indian History,* 76.
[127] Eaton, *Essays on Islam and Indian History,* 32.

generalized scale, Sufis self-identified as Muslims on a mystical path of Islam with the goal of communing with God. This communion occurs through complete annihilation of the human soul, which is achieved through love and devotion to God.[128] The word for Sufi, *ṣūf*, means literally "one who wears wool," and another grammatical form, *taṣawwuf*, means the phenomenon of mysticism.[129] Sufism arose in the eighth to tenth centuries of the Common Era (CE) and was loosely associated with the expansion and contraction of the Ghaznavid court across Persia, Khorasan, Transoxiana and the northwest of the Indian subcontinent. In contrast to Islam, Sufi philosophy believes one can have a direct experience with God. It has historically been thought that the mystical aspects of Sufism came from somewhere other than Islam, since it was assumed "that Islam was legalistic and intolerant" and thus would not have such blissful, mystical experiences in their religious roster.[130]

Of course, it is a little more complicated than that. There are multiple orders of Sufis that arose in different places and so were disaggregated in beliefs and practices. Regardless, they all shared similar monotheistic beliefs in which the legalistic Islamic path was seen to not quite go far enough in its devotion to God as it was still concerned with worldly pleasures and politics, which Sufis broadly opposed. Sufis, though not necessarily self-recognized as such until long after they first started writing, wrote about the need to have one-pointed attention on God without worldly distractions.[131] Thus, they led a more ascetic lifestyle, to varying degrees depending upon the order within which one practiced, and were additionally focused on practicing love for God.

---

[128] Marshall G.S. Hodgson, *The venture of Islam: conscience and history in a world civilization*, Vol. 1 (Chicago: University of Chicago Press, 1974), 393.
[129] L. Massington, et al. "Taṣawwuf," in *Encyclopaedia of Islam* 2nd Edition, Edited by: P. Bearman, Th. Bianquis, C.E. Bosworth, E. van Donzel, W.P. Heinrichs.
[130] Carl W. Ernst, "Sufism and Yoga According to Muhammad Ghawth," *Sufi* 29 (1996): 9.
[131] Annemarie Schimmel, *Mystical Dimensions of Islam* (The University of North Carolina Press, 1975): 46.

What specific religious beliefs and practices did Sufis and yogis share? As mentioned earlier, both groups practiced asceticism to varying degrees, and the general goal was to become liberated from the world. For yogis, liberation broadly means a "release from time and space and causality," though of course different schools of yoga treat that differently, as we saw in section one.[132] For Sufis, this idea of liberation existed but it was not the final goal, rather one step towards it. The final goal for most Sufi orders is *fanā*, literally "annihilation" of the self through "union or communion with God," which can only be achieved after experiencing "purity of heart," which Zaehner (1960) claims corresponds to mokṣa.[133] The additional difference, and perhaps the most important, is love. While there is a form of yoga called *bhakti* yoga that includes love for the divine, that is not the form of yoga the Sufis would have first encountered in the Indo-Gangetic plains. Rather, it seems most of the texts in this section are addressing Nāth yogis, who have tantric associations and are known for their supernatural powers. Importantly, there was no self-identified, unified, or organized order of Nāth yogis before the seventeenth century, so the title itself is not found in the Persian or Sanskrit literature we are addressing here. However, it is recognized that there were a few traditions of yogic practices that were later collected under the "Nāth Sampradāya" title and were all only referred to as "Yogis" or "Jogis" in the texts we are analyzing.[134] Additionally, the different *sampradāyas* (traditions) of yogis are known to have spent time with each other, so there are not necessarily clear distinctions between

---

[132] Robert Charles Zaehner, *Hindu and Muslim Mysticism* (Schocken Books, 1960), 6.
[133] Zaehner, *Hindu and Muslim Mysticism,* 7. The Shaṭṭarī Sufi order, from which Ghawth Gwaliari and Rājgīrī, two of the authors examined in this section, does not believe in fanā [see Khan Sahib Khaja Khan, *Studies in Tasawwuf* (INdia: Idarah-I Adabiyat-I Delli, 1923)].
[134] Daniela Bevilacqua, "Introduction," *The Power of the Nāth Yogis: Yogic Charisma, Political Influence and Social Authority*, ed. Daniela Bevilacqua and Eloisa Stuparich (Amsterdam University Press, 2022), 11.

each group.[135] Regardless, the largest group in the area were the Nāth yogis, so I will primarily focus on scholarship about them.

Nāth yogis believe in "occult powers that culminate in immortality and deification," and include alchemical "transmutation of sexual fluids into elixir."[136] Many of the texts we are examining here mock these sorts of powers, and yet the first known medieval Bengali description of a Sufi saint includes much the same descriptions, such as curing illness and reading minds.[137] If the Bengali description did not specifically call the person a Sufi, they may well have been assumed to be a yogi since that is what the Bengali people would have been more familiar with. While the Sufis doubted the yogis' ability to perform these supernatural feats, they shared many of the practices which supposedly helped attain the abilities, such as breath control and meditation.[138]

Due to the similarity in practices, some scholars in the past suggested that Sufism was emerged from a synthesis of Islam and yogic practices. While some Sufis likely did have access to yogic thinking as early as the eighth century CE, recent scholarship, such as Eaton (2000), Maas and Verdon (2018), and Ernst (2005), shows that some of the yogic practices were absorbed into Sufi practices rather than used as a source of religious or philosophical knowledge.[139] It is important to keep in mind that there were many schools of Sufis and the Sufis that were primarily South Asian had different catalysts and trajectories than those outside of South Asia. I would suggest that it is more likely that the practices had much overlap anyway, being that both Sufis and yogis practice asceticism, and so it may not be possible to distinguish

---

[135] Daniela Bevilacqua, "Let the Sādhus Talk: Ascetic Understanding of Haṭha Yoga and Yogāsanas," *Religions of South Asia* 11, no. 2-3 (2017): 185-186.
[136] Gordon Djurdjevic, *Masters of Magical Powers: The Nāth Siddhas in the Light of Esoteric Notions* (2005), ii.
[137] Eaton, *Essays on Islam and Indian History,* 32.
[138] James Mallinson, "*The Original Goraksaśataka*," *Yoga in Practice*, ed. Gordon White (Princeton University Press, 2012), 258.
[139] Mallinson, "*The Original Goraksaśataka*," 258.

what were strictly "yoga" versus "Sufi" practices. Each tradition has its own canon so to speak, but both rely primarily on the teacher-student transmission of practice (*paramparā* in the yogic context and *silsilā* in the Sufi context). While there are many texts that consider themselves part of a larger yoga school of philosophy, some of which were examined in the first section, each sampradāya has its own texts and may consider some of the other yoga texts as not part of the larger canon. As Bevilacqua (2017) shows, even modern yogis do not consider texts to be a good mode of teaching, but instead are for the purpose of people who cannot practice yoga all the time. In other words, canonical yogic texts are intended for householders, not dedicated yogis.[140] Partially, this is due to the fact that the practices are supposed to be secret and kept within the sampradāya only.[141] There are of course many texts that call themselves part of the yoga canon, but there are so many sampradāyas it is difficult to find clear unity between them.

Likewise, there is no official Sufi canon that is meant to teach Sufism; rather, there is much poetry and literature and historiographies, but no official text that teaches the tradition in any substantial way because initiates are supposed to learn from a proper teacher. Thus, even the texts closest to being instructional stop short of describing ecstatic states or the more esoteric experiences that dedicated practitioners achieve. This lack of description could partially be due to the fact that it is not possible to really convey these experiences in words, but it is also due to the covetousness of the tradition's practices remaining within the silsila, at least to some orders.[142] Despite neither yogis or Sufis finding writing to be an adequate mode of transmitting

---

[140] Bevilacqua, "Let the Sādhus Talk: Ascetic Understanding of Haṭha Yoga and Yogāsanas," 190.
[141] See [Bevilacqua, "Let the Sādhus Talk: Ascetic Understanding of Haṭha Yoga and Yogāsanas," 191] for the yogic context and [Eaton, *Essays on Islam and Indian History*. (Cambridge: Oxford University Press, 2000), 118] for the Sufi context.
[142] Schimmel, *Mystical Dimensions of Islam,* 59.

their practices and beliefs, the Sufis in particular wrote quite a lot and have left a trail of texts that exemplify their understanding of the world around them.

2.1.4 Arabic, Persian, or Other?

While the earliest Muslims in South Asia primarily spoke Arabic, the people that already inhabited the Indo-Gangetic Plains within which the Muslims were settling primarily spoke an early form of Hindi and other vernaculars.[143] What was unique to this location is that they used a separate language from what they spoke at home—Sanskrit—specifically for courtly affairs and the purposes of various knowledge systems, which includes politics, sciences, religious doctrines, grammar, ritual performances, and literature.[144] Yoga texts, too, were most often written in Sanskrit. The almost-exclusive use of a language for literary purposes and cultural identity was a new experience for the Muslim people. In other words, the Sanskrit language was used to transcend the physical boundaries of local languages for the purpose of transmitting religious, scientific, and cultural values. Persian developed later than Sanskrit, beginning around the seventh century in the Iranian Plateau, but was used in much the same way for the same purposes. Alongside and in place of Sanskrit, Persian became used in the courtly culture of the Delhi Sultanate between the tenth and twelfth centuries.[145] The writing styles that emerged shared characteristics of Sanskrit epics but added their own unique imagery and descriptions based on the authors' non-Sanskritic cultural and religious milieu.[146] Persian developed various

[143] A prakrit is a language that is spoken for everyday purposes in daily life. The distinction between Sanskrit as a cosmopolitan language that transcended borders and local languages that were unique to particular places and things was developed by Sheldon Pollock (2006).
[144] Sheldon Pollock, *The Language of the Gods in the World of Men* (Oakland: University of California Press, 2006).
[145] Daud Ali, *Courtly Culture and Political Life in Early Medieval India* (United Kingdom: Cambridge University Press, 2006), 266.
[146] Nile Green, editor, *The Persianate World: The Frontiers of a Eurasian Lingua Franca.* (Oakland: University of California Press, 2019) DOI: https://doi.org/10.1525/luminos, 64.

literary forms unique to its language and use.[147] It was in the eleventh century that Sufis started using Persian to record their philosophies, histories, and poetic expressions, and Persian quickly became the primary mode of Sufi authorship.[148] One of the genres particular to Sufis was *malfūẓ*, "the recounting of conversations of spiritually enlightened figures."[149] The similar use-cases of Persian and Sanskrit is another reason to examine the Sufi depictions of yogis, rather than another group, because they use similar modes of expression, adding a linguistic layer of understanding in addition to the religious beliefs and practices.

2.2 Al-Bīrūnī's *Kitāb Bātanjal* (The Yogasūtras of Patañjali)

Abū Rayḥān al-Bīrūnī was a scientist and polymath who translated *Pātañjali's Yogasūtras* (PYS) into Arabic in the late 1020s CE, which he titled *Kitāb Bātanjali al-Hindī* (KB). Al-Bīrūnī was native to the city-state of Khwārazm in modern-day Turkmenistan and Uzbekistan, and his first language was Khwārazmian, not Arabic. The purpose of his arrival in the Ghaznavid court after the city was annexed in 1017 CE is debated, but what is important is that he spent over a decade in the Punjab and surrounding regions learning the local languages, cultures, and beliefs before compiling his translation.[150] This led to the creation of a new methodology for comparative religious study by allowing the texts and pandits to speak for themselves rather than try to force some kind of universalism or fit them into Muslim (or other) categories.

---

[147] Muzaffar Alam, "Persian in Precolonial Hindustan," in *Literary Cultures in History*, ed. Sheldon Pollock (Oakland: University of California Press, 2003), 133.
[148] Shahzad Bashir, "The Persian World: A Literary Language in Motion," *Teaching the Global Middle Ages*, ed. Geraldine Heng (Modern Language Association of America, 2022), 119.
[149] Alam, "Persian in Precolonial Hindustan," 135.
[150] David Gordon White. "Foreword," *The Yoga Sūtras of Patañjali by Abū Rayḥān al-Bīrūnī*, trans. by Mario Kozah (New York: New York University Press, 2022), x-xiv.

Al-Bīrūnī had direct contact with Abū Alī al-Ḥusayn Ibn Sīnā, one of the primary "founding figures of the Arabic philosophical tradition," which provides clear evidence into the philosophical and scientific milieu of the time, namely the Peripatetic school of natural philosophy from which al-Bīrūnī clearly distinguishes himself.[151] He also had access to a multitude of sources from all over the contacted world on topics ranging from medicine to astronomy to political treatises and poetry. Needless to say, he had a solid basis for his exploration of these wide-ranging topics as he encountered new ways of thinking about them in the Ghaznavid courts.

Over the course of his stay in the Ghaznavid courts, beginning in 1017, al-Bīrūnī learned Sanskrit and had contact with various local pandits. In 1030, not long after he completed the KB, al-Bīrūnī composed another work titled *Tarik al-Hind* (*Hind*, henceforth) which was essentially an encyclopedia of the philosophies and sciences he encountered in India. In the introduction to Hind, he states that he hopes people read this text instead of his earlier texts, including the KB, because his understanding of Sanskrit had improved and he had more access to relevant scholars so he feared the earlier translations were not as accurate as they ought to be.[152] Frankly, al-Bīrūnī had a remarkable understanding of how writers before him tended to "produce the arguments of our antagonists in order to refute such of them as I believe to be in the wrong" and that he wanted to instead create "a simple historic record of facts."[153] While we examine his translation of the PYS, it is important to keep in mind this goal and so assume that any errors he makes are due to what knowledge and resources he had access to rather than a purposeful

[151] For a more in-depth exploration of this context, see Kozah (2015), *The Birth of Indology as an Islamic Science: Al-Bīrūnī's Treatise on Yoga Psychology*.
[152] Abū Rayḥān al-Bīrūnī, *Alberuni's India*, trans. Edward C. Sachau (London: Kegan Paul, Trench, Trubner & Co Ltd, 1910), 7-8.
[153] Al-Bīrūnī, *Alberuni's India*, 7.

misrepresentation. This claim about earlier scholars marks a clear distinction in the way al-Bīrūnī conceptualized the "other"; earlier scholars had either ignored the religions of India or mocked them, indicating that they clearly positioned them as an "other"—i.e., in opposition to their own set of beliefs and practices, and clearly lesser-than. Al-Bīrūnī on the other hand approached Indian religions with acceptance and desire to understand rather than alienate, even though he stated he believed they were not always correct and even heretical.

It should be noted that the KB was not simply a direct translation, but al-Bīrūnī also included at least one commentary.[154] He presents the PYS in dialogic style rather than the original poetic sūtra style, which allows him to both explain the philosophy as well as "correctively revise,"[155] to borrow Kozah's terminology, the style to make it more accessible to people unfamiliar with the Sanskrit commentarial tradition.[156] He notes that the PYS text he had access to was in meter with separate commentaries that heavily relied on grammar, etymology, and other areas that used more scholarly language and vernacular terms that he thought unnecessary for his intended Arabic-reading audience.[157]

When al-Bīrūnī was traveling in India, the PYS was still popular and relatively well-respected. There were of course tensions between religious communities with different beliefs (see the commentaries by Śrīvaiṣṇava theologian Rāmānuja and Jain philosopher Hemacandra for examples), but it was not until the twelfth century that commentaries on—and thus the influence of—the Yogasūtras petered out.[158] Thus, it is not as though al-Bīrūnī had access to some obscure, secret ancient text, but rather PYS was part of the larger philosophical narrative in

---

[154] Abū Rayḥān Al-Bīrūnī. *Kitāb Bātanjal (The Yoga Sūtras of Patañjali)*. Translated by Mario Kozah. New York University Press, 2020. pg xiv-xv

[155] Al-Bīrūnī, *Kitāb Bātanjal*, 4.

[156] Kozah, Mario. *The Birth of Indology as an Islamic Science,* Pg 85.

[157] Al-Bīrūnī, *Kitāb Bātanjal*, 4. The PYS we have access to today is not in meter, so this suggests it may not have been the same text that he had access to.

[158] White, "Foreword," xiv.

India at the time. Additionally, it seems that he had access primarily to non-dualist interpretations of yoga, which were counter to the dualist teachings in PYS.[159] He does not make it clear which commentaries he was translating, though there are some hints. As White notes, al-Bīrūnī suggests he will make an exposition "in the style of Hiraṇyagarbha" before he begins the translation of the actual text, which is really unusual because there is no actual evidence of a person writing by the name Hiraṇyagarbha, though there are later commentaries that make reference to an apparently lost text by the name *Hiraṇyagarbha Yogaśāstra.*[160] If indeed there was such a text, it is plausible that al-Bīrūnī had access to it and it may be the source of his translation, as it is unclear what other author or text he is imitating the style of. Further research is needed to determine who or what Hiraṇyagarbha was in this context as a preliminary search did not return useful results, but that is outside the scope of this thesis.[161]

The exact sources of who and what al-Bīrūnī had access to in India are unclear but the impacts he left on scholarship and literature were significant. It has been claimed that he was the first to systematically categorize what he considered "Indian" beliefs into one religion, namely in the *Hind.*[162] To accomplish this, he actually relied heavily upon his translation and understanding of PYS to claim it is the "Holy Book" of Indians.[163] He also claims that transmigration of the soul ("metempsychosis") is the defining belief of all "Indian religion."[164] While these are vast

---

[159] White, "Foreword," xvii.
[160] White, "Foreword," xvii.
[161] There is mention of Hiraṇyagarbha in the *Mahābhārata*, specifically as Brahman or Viṣṇu (Apte Practical Sanskrit-English Dictionary). The term also comes up as being the creator of yoga, as in the original teacher, with the suggestion that Patañjali compiled the works of Hiraṇyagarbha into one concise treatise (See: Nalinī Śuklā, *Pātañjala-Yogasūtra kā vivecanātmaka evaṃ tulanātmaka adhyayana* (Śaktiyogāśrama, 1975)). Still, none of these explanations are particularly helpful without consulting al-Biruni's original Arabic and analyzing what commentaries and yoga texts are known to have been accessible by him. One such commentary is written or commissioned by King Bhoja called *Rājamārtaṇḍa*; Bhoja is mentioned in al-Bīrūnī's *Hind* so it may have been accessible as he was at least aware of its commissioner (Al-Bīrūnī, *Alberuni's India* 1, 300).
[162] Kozah, *The Birth of Indology as an Islamic Science,* 1.
[163] Kozah, *The Birth of Indology as an Islamic Science,* 2.
[164] Kozah, *The Birth of Indology as an Islamic Science,* 2.

simplifications, the purpose, as al-Bīrūnī states it, was to make "Indian religion" more accessible to the Muslim reader of al-Bīrūnī's work. While this may make us inclined to believe his writing is too biased to be useful, or somehow incorrect, his methodology has been shown to be sound in that he chose to engage with Indian thought as it was rather than as he thought it should be, where scholars before him had ignored it completely or belittled it, and scholars after him did not seem to appreciate his open-minded stance.[165] Additionally, where something was unclear, rather than try to finagle an explanation into his translation, he simply quoted the direct source and then expounded upon it. Thus, this is al-Bīrūnī's creation of the new methodology for comparative religious studies.

To exemplify how al-Bīrūnī was conducting his comparative study, we can look at some of the rare places in his text where he conflates his own understanding of religious ideas with the beliefs in PYS. An interesting and informative distinction is the section where, in al-Bīrūnī's translation, a questioner asks Patañjali if there is "a path to liberation other than the two paths of practice and dispassion."[166] Patañjali answers that yes, there is the opportunity to achieve liberation through devotion.[167] The questioner asks further, "Who is this object of devotion who grants felicity?" The answer of God is given, who is described as having primacy and unity, no need for action, free from thoughts, transcends opposites, and is omniscient.[168] This is a distinct difference from the copies we have of Patañjali's text, wherein the *īśvara* (god) is the Lord of Yoga—a perfect example of a yoga practitioner who has achieved true liberation—rather than "a creator god who grants grace."[169] In fact, the entire section on God in al-Bīrūnī's translation is

---

[165] Lawrence, "Al-Bīrūnī's Approach to the Comparative Study of Indian Culture," 150.
[166] Al-Bīrūnī, *Kitāb Bātanjal.* Section 11.1
[167] Ibid. Section 11.2
[168] Section 12.2
[169] Stoler Miller, *Yoga: Discipline of Freedom*, 32.

longer than in Patañjali's, the former going on from 11.1 to 21.2 (twelve full verses), and the latter going from 23 to 27 (five full verses). Given that he likely had access to nondualist sources, it is possible that this description of a god that transcends opposites actually arises from the commentaries he was translating rather than his own Islamic philosophy, or perhaps that he was conflating the two. It would be useful in our understanding of al-Bīrūnī's "othering" if scholars could determine what commentaries he had access to.[170]

Another example of the ambiguity regarding whether al-Bīrūnī was superimposing his own mapping of these concepts or just working with commentators is when the KB discusses the corruptions of the mind. One of the examples for the ties of corruption is the things men do when lusting after women, such as bringing gifts, wearing perfume, and flirting. Another example given for the same corruption is a fixation with predicting one's own death.[171] The latter seems more a topic that Patañjali or a Sanskrit commentator might allude to rather than the former, though without reading the commentary from which he drew his translations, I cannot say for sure. While yogis are most often celibate, and so the idea of lust may be an accurate problem one would use as an example of the ties of corruption, it is not found in any version of PYS we have access to now.

In order to fully understand whether al-Bīrūnī was being true to his sources we need to determine exactly what those sources may be. As he notes in the *Hind*, he had access to documents from all over India and from various schools of thought, so it seems that he primarily gained his knowledge through study of primary texts (or commentaries thereof), unlike his

---

[170] Some work has been done on trying to source the commentaries and original texts al-Bīrūnī used. See [Ajay Mitra Shastri, "Sanskrit Literature known to al-Bīrūnī," *Indian Journal of the History of Science* 10, num. 2.] and [Noemie Verdon, "Bīrūnī as a source for the study of Indian culture and history." Presented at the International Seminar on Travelogue in JNU, Delhi, March 2012].
[171] Al-Bīrūnī, *Kitāb Bātanjal*, Section 27.6

predecessors who seemed to have only formed their theses based on oral accounts or direct experience, which was colored by their personal biases. According to al-Bīrūnī, earlier Islamicate scholars engaged in a belittling othering of the Indian beliefs and peoples, while al-Bīrūnī himself seems to have engaged more honestly with them, or at least tried to. If we consider othering in the colonial context, it is often derogatory and intended as a tool to simplify a group of people or beliefs, so it was easier to create narratives about the dynamics of power and societal development or progression (or lack thereof).[172] On the contrary, al-Bīrūnī, while explicitly claiming he did not share all the beliefs he was describing, attempted to examine the beliefs and sources he had from a non-biased perspective as quoted earlier in this section, thus narrowing the gap of the othering that occurred before him. It is of course possible that he was being disingenuous about his motives and was in fact constructing a narrative encouraged by the Ghaznavid court for which he worked, but without finding correspondence or evidence of these sorts of directives, I cannot say. His own scientific work was informed by the sciences he learned about in India. While he did collapse the various schools of belief and practices of the Indian subcontinent into one "Indian religion," he seemed to do this not as an attempt to create a dynamic of power or progression but rather as a way to make the landscape more accessible to his readers. I believe pinpointing this goal of his writing is important in looking at the bigger picture of the impacts of his methodologies and "othering" because his work was very intentional, and he was impressively self-aware about what he was doing and how. While no one can foresee the consequences of their scholarship, the fact that we still use al-Bīrūnī's texts shows us that his framing of the intellectual and religious landscape was not as problematic as his contemporary scholars might have us believe.

[172] Edward Said, *Orientalism*, (New York: Pantheon Books, 1978).

Thus, I am left with more questions than I have answers, that would be interesting to explore in later scholarship. These questions are: What texts did al-Bīrūnī have access to? PYS manuscripts, commentaries, etc. Who did al-Bīrūnī consult for his learning? What language did they communicate in? Did al-Bīrūnī receive specific instruction from the Ghaznavid court to complete this work? If so, for what purpose? If al-Bīrūnī did not receive direct instructions from the court to perform this translation, what was his goal? What specific wording did al-Bīrūnī use when speaking of yogis and India and the people he was working with? Since I cannot read the Perso-Arabic script (*naskh*) he wrote in, and I do not know Arabic, the exact words and meaning are unavailable to me without relying on transcriptions and translators who will choose their own wordage for various reasons and may or may not reflect al-Bīrūnī's intended meaning. How did other scholars and readers of al-Bīrūnī's texts respond to the content? Once there are answers to these questions, it will be possible to complete a new intellectual history of al-Bīrūnī and have a better understanding of how exactly he performed othering, not to mention how reliable his accounts of yogis (and other topics) are.

2.3 *Medieval Sufi Tales of Jogis*[173] translated by Simon Digby

Digby translated a collection of direct depictions of Sufi encounters of yogis composed in the twelfth to thirteenth centuries. Where exactly these tales came from is unclear, though some are from known collections. He also does not provide the originals from which he based his translations. Though these tales are in narrative form, they seem to be based on real encounters, though may be distorted interpretations of events rather than strictly factual retellings. While al-

[173] The transliteration of "yogi" is often "jogi" in the vernacular and Persianate context. I will use both interchangeably where appropriate.

Bīrūnī's text was non-fiction presented in dialogue, these tales are more fictitious and thus distinguishing between storytelling and fact is difficult. One way to frame the tales in this section is by looking at the broader historical context. The early twelfth century during which these tales began to be composed saw the beginning of Sultanate rule in the Indian subcontinent. The transition to this mode of governance was not always met with positivity by the people who were used to having a relatively decentralized society wherein they were mostly just accountable to their local governance units. Urban expansion, greater trade, and more use of money and taxes were significant shifts compared to pre-Sultanate rule.[174] The people living in the lands surrounding the garrison-towns in which the Sultans ruled were considered by the courts to be *mawās* (rebellious) up until the fourteenth century at least.[175] This tension was not just political, but also religious and cultural. Cultural practices such as the caste system and polytheism were trying to fit into this new Sultanate paradigm.

Digby states that, to the Muslims, there was a distinction "between universal and local" devotion that distinguished between Islamic power and a desire to sanctify the spiritual power of the locales within which they found themselves.[176] All of the tales Digby has translated here recognize a similarity between yogic practices and Sufi practices, which is a significant shift from al-Bīrūnī seeing the yoga described in his Kitāb Bātanjal as somehow separate from Islam. The stories in this collection of Sufi tales about jogis are direct examples of how these dynamics between universal and local, familiar and unfamiliar, may have played out, at least in the literary imagination. Overall, the Sufi Shaykhs do not seem to trust the jogis, their claims to supernatural powers, or overall ethics. While al-Bīrūnī's othering only one or two hundred years earlier was

[174] Irfan Habib, *Medieval India: The Study of a Civilization* (India: National Book Trust, 2007), 63-64.
[175] Habib, *Medieval India: The Study of a Civilization*, 57-58.
[176] Simon Digby, "To Ride a Tiger or a Wall: Strategies of Prestige in Indian Sufi Legend," *According to Tradition: Hagiographical Writing in India* (Harrassowitz Verlag, Wiesbaden, 1994), 99.

more considerate, the tides seem to have turned as far as how willing the Sufis were to entertain the belief systems of the jogis. While it is not realistic to extrapolate these stories to be representative of the greater feelings of the Sultanate rulers of the time, or the wider Muslim population at large, it is important to think about how the Sufi literature was being circulated to the people, who those people were, and what impact these depictions of yogis may have had on the dynamics between groups of people in the real world.

The stories in this collection are short and tend to depict one or two jogis in very specific settings, which makes it seem like these may be representative of events that were actually witnessed. The tone of these tales is one of general disdain and even belittling, much like what al-Bīrūnī claims to have seen in earlier scholars. Whether this is the tone intended in the original or overlaid by Digby's translation is hard to say, but the content itself generally supports this reading of the general tone, other than the second story which we will examine below.

The first story is of a jogi named Bālgundai. The jogi traveled far at the behest of his *guru* (*pīr* in Persian) to see Sayyīd Muhammad Gesūdarāz, a respected Shaykh, and to give him a gift. This theme of gifting speaks from two angles. First, there are many customs around gift-giving in South Asia over history.[177] It was common for people to give gifts to show fealty to the ruler, and rulers would gift land-grants and women to other rulers to secure political and religious treatises and patronage. Second, "many sufis expressed scorn for assured or regular gifts and land-grants."[178] If we look at this tale from the first angle, it seems the jogi Bālgundai was doing something appropriate and it was the Shaykh that was in the wrong for denying the gifts, as I will show in detail below. However, if we look at this tale from the second angle, it

[177] Maria Heim, *Theories of the Gift in South Asia: Hindu, Buddhist, and Jain Reflections on Dana* (New York: Routledge, 2004).
[178] Habib, *Medieval India: The Study of a Civilization*, 82.

could be that the Sufi author was aligning themselves with the Shaykh's court and thus the jogi giving the court a gift is as if they were giving the Sufis a gift and that could be seen as ultimate disrespect.

The first gift Bālgundai tried to give Gesūdarāz was alchemy, and when Gesūdarāz did not accept that, he tried to gift him a warning about the future. Again, Gesūdarāz did not accept it, so Bālgundai tried to gift him the ability to become invisible. When that was not accepted, Bālgundai tried to gift him the ability to "hold back" his sexual release. Again, he was rejected. Finally, Bālgundai tried to gift Gesūdarāz the ability to move things with his mind (telekinesis), but again was denied. Gesūdarāz then gifted Bālgundai a single coin and a pomegranate fruit, ultimately putting him to shame as the jogi could not deny these gifts without being disrespectful.

After Bālgundai leaves, the people of the court explain that Bālgundai was put to death many times but always reappeared. In other words, he was a powerful being who could defy death. However, it was explained that he had alchemy but not magic. The statement that he has no magic is an important critique of the yogis. To Sufis, magic is equivalent to miracles, and miracles are something only God can perform.[179] For a human to say they can perform magic, therefore, is the same as saying they can perform miracles, and that is blasphemous. Further description of Bālgundai describes him as wearing all white. One of the accounts of him was "seated in a posture of meditation with his two feet upon his thighs."[180] This is typical of a yogi aesthetic and so makes it even more clear to the reader that the person in the story who was

[179] Patton Burchett, "My Miracle Trumps Your Magic: Encounters With Yogīs in Sufi and Bhakti Hagiographical Literature," *Yoga Powers*, ed. Knut A. Jacobsen (Boston: Brill, 2012), 345-380: 350.
[180] "Medieval Sufi Tales of Jogis," *Wonder-Tales of South Asia: Translated from Hindi, Urdu, Nepali, and Persian.* Translated by Simon Digby. Oxford University Press, 2006. pg 225

ultimately in the wrong is the yogi and extends this criticism to all yogis by explicitly associating Bālgundai with the group to which he belongs.

The second story is difficult to decipher on its own because it is so short and does not give much description. However, it seems to be a retelling of a popular Nāth yogi legend regarding Gorakhnāth and his guru Matsyendra the founder of the Nāth yogi school. In the Nāth yogi legend, Matsyendra becomes a consort of a queen and Gorakhnāth convinces him to renounce the householder's life and return to the path of the yogi.[181] This tale originally functions as part of the Nāth teachings about the beginning of their lineage as well as enforcing renunciation as the ultimate path and also diverging from some of the more tantric practices regarding sexuality and ritual practiced beforehand. This tale is dated between the ninth and eleventh century.

The tale as told in Digby's selection of Sufi Tales tells it in a new way and depicts jogis as if they have no empathy. While the jogis' names are not given in the tale itself, the names do appear in the title. The Sufi version of the story is as follows. There were two jogis that were traveling together. One is a teacher (*Pīr*) and the other is his student (*Murīd*). They split ways and the teacher gets caught up in the material world, performing sexual acts, creating a family, and even becoming a ruler of a small village. He is a ruler for some time before the other finds him and convinces him to return to the proper path—that of a yogi. He does so but brings with him a son, which the student jogi claimed was a distraction to their practice. They end up killing the boy so they can focus on their practice of yoga.

This is a drastic variation from the original Nāth telling of the story. It is hard to say for sure what the story was trying to do since there is not much detail in the story itself, but it seems

---

[181] David N. Lorenzen, *Yogi Heroes and Poets: Histories and Legends of the Nāths* (Albany: State University of New York Press, 2011), 36.

on the surface to depict yogis as lacking empathy because the only reason they were bothered by the child was because he kept asking if he could stop meditating to relieve himself. Thinking in a Sufi context, where love is the most important facet of their beliefs, this story could also be showing that yogis lack love. Having said that, there are legends of great Sufis who claimed to be happy when their sons died before them so they could focus their love on God, and Abraham himself sacrificed his son.[182] So telling this Gorakhnāth story this way may actually shed a positive light on the yogis and the Nāth sampradāya in particular.

The third story is that in which a cat is the main character. The cat was originally owned by a jogi named Kamāl, but upon hearing a Shaykh give a discourse on an unspecified holy topic, it would not leave the Shaykh's company. Clearly, this is to indicate that even a cat can understand that Islam is superior to joga.

The fourth story is a contest between a jogi and a Shaykh, in which the jogi came to the Shaykh and challenged him to show any powers that the jogi would be unable to duplicate. The jogi shows that he can raise up into the air. The Shaykh says to God that he had gifted the jogi the ability to do this, someone who "is a stranger to Thee," so God should also bestow the ability upon the Shaykh.[183] The Shaykh was able to fly all around rather than just straight upwards, so the jogi declares that his own power is false and converts to Islam.

The fifth story is of a jogi who had a Philosopher's Stone and attempted to gift it to a Shaykh, but the Shaykh did not accept because he felt no need for material goods. Ultimately, the jogi recognizes the Shaykh's holiness and superiority and converts to Islam under his guidance. Here we have an example of gift giving again, as in the first story, but with less emphasis. The point here is that the jogi is on the wrong path and is only saved by Islam.

---

[182] Schimmel, *Mystical Dimensions of Islam*, 14; 36.
[183] "Medieval Sufi Tales of Jogis," 229

The sixth story is a general teaching that the alchemical and magical powers that jogis have are not what God wants, and when they try to give gifts of alchemy and magic to Shaykhs, the gifts should be ignored because they are trials by God through which He is testing their devotion and strength. People which possess these powers have "dark hearts" and "the graces and inspirations of God are no longer his lot."[184] This is an important distinction since, as we saw before, Sufis are often described as having the same powers as yogis but are given them by God's grace. In this case, Sufis are writing these tales and saying that these powers go against the path of God.

Overall, these tales paint yogis in a very negative light, as not only being wrong in their actions and abilities, but also actively trying to dissuade holy men from their own relation with God. This could be an attempt at showing that, while yogis and Sufis are similar in their practices, they are not the same. Indeed, they seem to be suggesting that the yogis cannot do what they claim and thus should not be given attention or respect, whereas the Sufis should. The second tale that is a retelling of the Gorakhnāth and Matsyendranāth tale is the most controversial as it is not necessarily a negative telling. Ultimately, without knowing who specifically wrote these stories and who the intended audience was, it is difficult to expand the analysis past the stories themselves and into the intellectual milieu in which they existed. If Sufis were writing these stories for other Sufis, they really seem more satirical than explicitly critical. If these stories are for a broader audience that are not already practicing Muslims, the stories come across as being more critical and demeaning. And if the stories are for the Shaykhs and Sultans, they are more precautionary and derogatory. It would be interesting to examine if other

[184] "Medieval Sufi Tales of Jogis," 233.

sources refer to these tales to see how they may have been received by contemporary audiences, and who those audiences were.

There is now evidence that the Nāth yogis had composed two texts with an intended audience of Muslims, called *Avali Silūk* and *Kāfir Bodh.* The manuscripts we have are from 1614 CE, so a few hundred years after these tales were composed. "[T]he Nāth yogis not only preached acceptance of Islamic beliefs and the continuation of Muslim obligatory practices but also had a desire to present their faith to Muslim communities as a continuation of Islam."[185] This is an incredibly important revelation as it suggests that these tales that Digby translated are not necessarily as fabricated as they may seem. Though these Nāth texts came after these tales, it is possible that the sentiment of cooperation had been there at the time of these tales also, so the yogis really were trying to win the acceptance of the Shaykhs and Sufis. Likewise, these tales seem to be strongly othering the yogis, and since these Nāth texts were officially composed long after these tales, it seems the othering on the part of the Sufis was ultimately unsuccessful, at least as far as its impact on the Nāth yogis at the time. This suggests that the audience was indeed not the yogis, but some other population.

2.4 Muhammad Ghawth Gwaliyari's *Bahr al-hayat* (The Ocean of Life)

Originally written in the fifteenth century, the *Bahr al-hayat* is a Persian translation of the Sanskrit text called *Amṛtakuṇḍa* by a Shaṭṭarī Sufi saint, Muhammad Ghawth Gwaliyari. It is important to note that he was a Shaṭṭarī Sufi because the Shaṭṭarī order "adopted yogic styles of devotion."[186] Thus, the depictions of yogis tended to be at least semi-favorable, and explains why

[185] Christine Marrewa-Karwoski. "The Erased 'Muslim' Texts of the Nath Sampradāy," *The Wire*, 2018. https://thewire.in/religion/the-erased-muslim-texts-of-the-nath-sampraday
[186] Kugle, Scott. "ʿAbdallāh Shaṭṭār," *Encyclopaedia of Islam*, volume three, Edited by Kate Fleet, Gudrun Krämer, Denis Matringe, John Nawas, Everett Rowson. 2013. http://dx.doi.org/10.1163/1573-3912_ei3_COM_23912

engaging with yoga texts and topics was acceptable, even if they were ambivalent.[187] The *Amṛtakuṇḍa* is a haṭha yoga text, typically attributed to the Nāth yogis, but the original text no longer exists. The text describes mantras, prāṇāyāma, āsana, and other spiritual practices found in the haṭha yoga tradition, painted in the fashion of making it accessible to Muslim readership.

Scattered throughout are quotes directly from the *Qur'an*. Since the quotes are at the end of the sentence, rather than a sentence on their own, it seems that Gwaliyari was reconciling the narrative descriptions with a saying from the Qur'an, thus lending authority to them. Despite this creative adaptation we see all through the text, section four compares terms directly rather than trying to strictly translate them: "In their technical terms they call recollection (*dhikr*) practice (*karma*), and they call asceticism and abstemiousness *dharma*. Their piety (*taqwa*)..."[188] Since not all the comparisons are just in brackets, it is clear that Ghawth Gwaliyari's text itself was doing this comparison, and it was not the English translator doing so. It would be interesting to study if these terms are truly equivalent or that is a superposition by Ghawth Gwaliyari as well. Without speaking to a Persian or Muslim scholar, and only consulting dictionaries, we can simply compare these terms.

Dhikr is a form of oral meditation or prayer in which one focuses on Allah.[189] Karma, in contrast, is literally translated as "action," though often means a sort of ritual action or discipline, so the translation here of practice is not incorrect. Though, if it originally meant an oral form of meditation or prayer in the *Amṛtakuṇḍa* is hard to say without analyzing the source text. There are existing translations into various languages, so an inter-manuscript study might shed light on this.

---

[187] Carl W. Ernst, "Sufism and Yoga According to Muhammad Ghawth," Sufi. Issue 29, 1996. pg 10.
[188] Ghawth Gwaliyari, Muhammad. *Bahr al-hayat (The Ocean of Life)*. Chapter 4, translated by Carl W. Ernst.
[189] L. Gardet, "Dhikr," *Encyclopaedia of Islam*, Second Edition, ed. P. Bearman, Th. Bianquis, C.E. Bosworth, E. van Donzel, W.P. Heinrichs, 2012.

Dharma is a very difficult term to translate to English. In the context of yogic texts, it is often meant to imply a sort of proper life path; "to follow your dharma" is a saying that we find often. For this text to compare it to asceticism, then, is not incorrect in this context, though may be a simplification, as asceticism is only one aspect of the yogic life path.

Taqwa as piety has an interesting connotation. According to the Brill Encyclopedia, taqwa has a connotation of fearing God. Yoga sampradāyas writ large do not believe in God in the universalized Abrahamic sense and fearing God is not really part of their narrative or beliefs.[190] While an individual yogi may have a personal god towards which they experience fear, yoga in general does not teach this sort of practice or belief.

Despite this translation overwriting their own religious and philosophical interpretations into the above terms, Gwaliyari still goes on to describe the physical and embodied practices as they are likely originally found in the Sanskrit text. This is because the Muslim mystics at the time could recognize the similarity between the poses and breathing practices of the yogis and their own.[191] They also had a fascination with "Islamizing" the meditation practices, in other words fitting the yogic practices into an Islamic paradigm, probably because they found them useful tools for achieving a connection with God without worldly distractions.[192] But the translations of these yogic texts tend to end by saying something about how the subject is ultimately a waste of time.[193] An example of this is any mention in the original text of associating *cakra* meditation with goddesses is described in this translation as "imagination," thus making it clear that the religious connotations were not compatible, nor giving them any real attention.[194]

---

[190] L. Lewisohn, "Taḳwā," *Encyclopaedia of Islam*, Second Edition, ed. P. Bearman, Th. Bianquis, C.E. Bosworth, E. van Donzel, W.P. Heinrichs, 2012.
[191] Ernst, "Sufism and Yoga According to Muhammad Ghawth," 10.
[192] Ernst, "A Fourteenth Century Persian Account of Breath Control and Meditation," 133.
[193] Ernst, "A Fourteenth Century Persian Account of Breath Control and Meditation," 134.
[194] Ernst, "A Fourteenth Century Persian Account of Breath Control and Meditation," 134.

Partly, this dismissal could be due to the Sufis' desire to maintain a closeness with the power of the royal courts. By positioning themselves against the jogis and purportedly proving the jogis are wrong or their practice is incomplete, the Sufis maintain a narrative about being a more powerful and thus useful ally of the courts. It was during the fourteenth century that "Sufi ideas began to penetrate the political sphere" so it is clear that they had political influence which could be beneficial to their orders in the sense of receiving land grants or other forms of patronage.[195]

2.5 Rājgīrī's *Madhumālatī*

Rājgīrī's text is not didactic in the way that the *Bahr al-hayat* or *Kitāb Bātanjal* are. Composed in 1545 by a Shaṭṭarī Sufi, the *Madhumālatī* follows much of the formulaic poetic elements from Sanskrit literature and simultaneously uses the spiritual quest model of Sufi romances, which makes it a unique text in the genre. While written in Persian, the Sanskrit formulaic elements include that of "*rasa* or the idea of sympathetic response as the cornerstone of their aesthetic agenda."[196] Looking at particular verses, we will see how the rasa is meant to display the practice of yoga as a means to overcoming the turning troubles in the mind—in this case, love.

The *Madhumālatī* shows the ascetic yogic life in relatively positive terms. The story itself is of a Prince who falls madly in love with someone named Madhumālatī. The lovers are separated which causes the Prince such pain and sorrow that he gives everything up to become a yogi and wander indefinitely. There is a very vivid description of what he looks like in this transformation:

[195] Blain Auer, *In the Mirror of Persian Kings* (Cambridge University Press, 2021), 139.
[196] Behl and Doniger, *Love's Subtle Magic*, 1.

"So acute was the pain of separation
he could not control himself.
He asked for a begging bowl
and a yogi's staff and crutch.
He marked his forehead with a circle,
smeared his body with ashes,
and hung shining earrings in both his ears.
He took his drinking cup firmly in hand,
and tightened the strings of his ascetic's viol.
Letting down his matted locks, he donned the patched
cloak and the girdle of rope.
With loincloth tied around his waist, the Prince took
the guise of a Gorakh yogi."[197]

This is a pretty standard description of a yogi even today. The fact that it specifically names him as a Gorakh yogi is intriguing, since this makes him of the denomination of Gorakh Nāth yogis of Northern India, which was the group of yogis most familiar to Persian-speaking and Sufi people, as we have already seen in this section. This suggests that the Sufi poets, or at the very least *this* Sufi poet—Rājgīrī—recognized the Nāth yogis as a distinct group that were in conversation with his Sufi order, and as we saw with the Medieval Sufi Tales by Digby above, the Nāths likely agreed.[198]

Essentially, this story is showing that being a yogi is alright, though it is not the ideal path, and it is only one step in the path towards attaining true closeness with God. It was not that the Prince was a yogi that saved his life, it was his one-pointed attention to love, and asceticism was what allowed him to focus on it. The object of love in these stories is often a stand-in for God, and the lover the stand-in for the devotee. The Prince, in this case the devotee, was so absorbed in his love for Madhumālatī, the stand-in for God, that he forgot all else. Fortune and

[197] Shaikh Mir Sayyid Manjhan Rājgīrī, *Madhumālatī: An Indian Sufi Romance.* Tran. Aditya Behl and Simon Weightman (Oxford World Classics, 2000), verse 172, pg 72.
[198] Marrewa-Karwoski, "The Erased 'Muslim' Texts of the Nath Sampradāy."

life itself meant nothing to him as long as he could attain union with Madhumālatī. Becoming a yogi allowed him to remove attachments to the material plane, which was a step towards this union, but it seems that it was not what he *chose* to do, but that it happened naturally due to his absorption. A line from the story reads: "If he gained perfection on the path of yoga,/he might yet meet his beloved again./ Through a vision of the Guru love is born,/ and the viol sounds the mystic note of absorption."[199] Thus, it could be argued that people who choose the path of asceticism for the sake of asceticism are still wrong, because it is really the vision of the Guru, i.e. Madhumālatī, that real love and absorption comes. As the story winds up, the Prince achieves all the material goods yet again, once he has truly found his love, leaving behind the life of the ascetic that was merely a stepping stone on the journey of finding love—i.e., finding God. It is important to note that he attains all the material goods again, since even Sufis do not normally feel that material goods are of any use. Thus, it is possible that his attaining them in this story is an example to showing that once you attain true love for God, it does not matter what material goods you have as you are not interested in them.

Another theme this story plays with in regard to yogis is that of engaging in sexual acts. Sexual union comes up twice as a simile. Love is clearly the dominant emotion running through this work, though one could argue that the feeling (*rasa*) portrayed in this first instance is that of wonder, another of the eight rasas used in Sanskrit and Persian poetics.[200] The first instance is when the Prince fell asleep: "Sleep seized his eyelids which had stayed apart./ Like yogis who practice sexual union,/ or parted lovers, his lashes came together."[201] The second instance is when nymphs are speaking of the Prince and Madhumālatī: "To look upon them is to taste the

---

[199] Rājgīrī, *Madhumālatī: An Indian Sufi Romance,* verse 174, pg 73.
[200] Ananta Charan Sukla, "Indian Intermedial Poetics: The Sanskrit Rasa-Dhvani Theory," *Cultura: International Journal of Philosophy of Culture and Axiology* 13, no. 2 (2016), 14.
[201] Sukla, "Indian Intermedial Poetics: The Sanskrit Rasa-Dhvani Theory," verse 65, pg 28.

joy/ of yogis in the state of mystical union."[202] The distinction of sexual union and mystical union is unusual because in Sufism one often is representative of the other.[203] The explicit instance of sexual union is shown in a positive light: that of falling into "sweet sleep" of "the greatest comfort."[204] This has both the connotation of love and wonder which are considered to be positive *rasa*s. Thus, Rājgīrī intentionally portrayed yogis in a favorable light, even if it did stop before claiming they could achieve true union without the fundamental aspect of love for the divine that was so prevalent in Sufi practice and belief. It is clear that Rājgīrī's othering is far less distinct than the position taken by earlier Sufi writers. In fact, though the Prince is not a Sufi himself, the fact that he could be a yogi *and* a practicing Sufi is groundbreaking and a good place to end this section as the dynamic seems to have come full circle, from al-Bīrūnī first conceptualizing the yogis as alien and even opposed to Islamic philosophy to five-hundred years later when Rājgīrī accepts the path of a yogi as something fully compatible with the path of a Sufi.

2.6 Conclusions: Early Islamicate Engagements

It is clear through these examples that the Sufis were grappling with how to understand and live alongside the Nāth yogis over many generations. It is not quite possible to separate these people into two distinct groups—Sufis and Yogis—quite so clearly but for the purposes of this exploration into the depictions of the other, it served to show that writ large, the Sufis saw the yogis as inferior to themselves, or at least incomplete, despite their similarities in practice. The overall feeling of the depictions slowly became more hospitable over time. We saw in the *Kitāb*

---

[202] Sukla, "Indian Intermedial Poetics: The Sanskrit Rasa-Dhvani Theory," verse 72, pg 31.
[203] Valerie J. Hoffman-Ladd, "Mysticism and Sexuality in Sufi Thought and Life," *Mystics Quarterly* 18, no. 3 (September 1992), 83.
[204] Rājgīrī, *Madhumālatī: An Indian Sufi Romance*, verse 65, pg 28.

Bātanjal an attempt to understand the yogic philosophy in a way compatible with Islamic belief systems and vocabulary while shifting away from the disdain towards "Indian religions" by earlier Muslim writers. In the Medieval Sufi Tales, however, we saw an attempt to situate yogis as less than the Shaykhs and Sufis in general, and clearly vying for their approval. Though it seems that there may be some further examination into the second story that retells the Nāth legend to determine if it is in fact intended to show the yogis as unempathetic and inferior. In the *Bahr al-hayat* we saw a similar approach as the *Kitāb Bātanjal* to retain the physical practices that echoed Sufi practices and even to absorb them into the Sufi practices, but a complete shrugging-off of any religious connotation or further significance. Lastly, in the *Madhumālatī*, we saw a more favorable depiction of yoga, though it still subordinated yogis to less than the true path to achieve union with God.

Overall, it seems correct that, as Digby claimed, Muslims local to northern India were trying to find a connection to the land and place and found the closest equivalent to their own beliefs and practices in the Nāth yogis. While the Sufis did not appear to see the yogis as some other religion in the sense of othering we so often see today—the lines were not so distinctly drawn—it is clear that they recognized a familiarity that threatened their own political power and had to decide how to live alongside this group. Whether this was a successful amalgamation of two distinct groups of people and practices is debatable and would require an entirely different study, but the gradual creation of the Persian language that absorbed Sanskrit poetic features and explicitly conversed with the local traditions shows that the attempt was at least made to find similarities and differences, and perhaps live more successfully alongside each other while fomenting their own unique cultures and belief systems.

3 Sanskrit Perspectives of Yoga

3.1 Introduction

Philosophy and poetry have often been considered separate and incompatible. Philosophy is how we conceptualize reality; poetry, on the other hand, is considered to exist in the imaginative realm. While some scholars and poets argue against the validity of examining philosophy within poetry, many poets of pre-modern India included philosophy and religion by necessity. As Sarkar (1985) argues, both *vyutpatti* (scholarship, learning) and *pratibhā* (imagination), "are essential to the making of a poet" for without intellect, the aesthetic sense of poetry would be simply empty.[205] These poets often dealt with subject matter that was by its very nature inherently philosophical—as in, theorizing about the meaning of life and reality itself. Even images of love were often caricatured by divine figures who represented different aspects of reality. Thus, philosophy and religion were such large motifs throughout society that it was seemingly impossible to remove them from the production of great epic literature. Indeed, poetry speaks to the human experience, embellishing it with *rasa* (feelings) and *alaṃkāra* (ornamentation) in such a way as to make the seeming mundanity of life less mundane. Excluding philosophy and religion from poetry would miss a large piece of the fabric of everyday life—especially in India, where culture, religion, and philosophy are intricately woven together.

It was not just poets who incorporated philosophy, but also playwrights. Most folktales also included philosophical topics. Many premodern stories worldwide grapple with the meaning of life and the human condition, whether overtly or otherwise. In Sanskrit kāvya, we see this in

[205] Ranajit Sarkar, *In Search of Kālīdāsa's Thought-World: A Study of Kumārasaṃbhava* (Lucknow: Akhila Bharatiya Sanskrit Parishad, 1985), 3.

the extreme, where poets and playwrights included direct quotes from philosophical treatises or religious rituals. Rather than take away from the aesthetic flavour of the written work, this often added to it—if it was done skillfully. All four texts I examine in this section skillfully deal with yoga philosophy and incorporate it into the greater aesthetic work. Kālidāsa in his *Kumārasambhava* (c. 300-400 CE), and Māgha in his *Śiśupālavadha* (c. 600-700 CE) both wrote poems that dealt directly with yoga philosophy; Kālidāsa included extant descriptions of yoga philosophy and practice throughout the poem. Māgha was more subtle about it by paraphrasing or quoting passages from prominent yoga texts, though not blatantly stating it as such. Kṛṣṇamiśra's topic in his *Prabodhacandrodaya* (c. 1000-1100 CE) was overtly philosophical, comparing the religions and their arguments throughout. And the Vetāla tales from the *Vetālapañcavimśati* (c. 900-1300 CE), while diverse in their array of stories and topics, included some commentary on the behaviour and appearance of yogis. What these all have in common is that they are not philosophical texts in and of themselves, as in they do not try to make a case in favour or against any way of thinking about the world, but rather they include the topics to add life to their words and scenes.

While the stories do not try to be overtly philosophical for the sake of philosophy, each author would have written them with an agenda in mind. Each has a slightly different agenda, of course, and it is within an examination of these agendas that we can start to see what the poet's own thoughts might have been. Other scholars have tired over attempts to glean the poet's own feelings from their texts, and I personally believe it is a futile effort. An author does not *necessarily* write for the sake of their own ideas. Rather, they could be composing something on request of a patron, for a particular audience, as an obligation to their Sanskrit education, ritual motivations, or simply to make money. Remember, these writers are not philosophers—they are poets and playwrights and storytellers. Their mission is not to convince the reader of a philosophical or religious set of ideas. Their mission is to entertain the reader, bring beauty into daily life, and tell exciting stories. Any attempt at interacting with philosophy is secondary, otherwise they would be writing a philosophical text instead of a poem. Pollock (2001) agrees: "According to Sanskrit literary theory … one does not ultimately *learn* anything specific to the reading of Sanskrit literature" itself, since that is the domain of *śāstra* (treatise).[206]

Having said that, there is of course the possibility that a teacher is writing in such a manner that a student would find it more interesting. Imagine being a teacher whose student is brilliant but hates the scriptures because he finds them boring. You still must teach him, so you find a way to teach that will be better received. Thus, you come up with the idea to write a poem or a play that would be entertaining while still imparting the values and teachings you want the student to learn. Of course, this is a possibility that we cannot overlook, but I argue that it is unusual in the broad overview of poetry and literature writ large, especially in the context of yoga philosophy and practice. Most depictions we see of yoga philosophy or yogis are a minute part of the overall work, so it cannot be taken as an instructive text. I will, however, try to determine if it may be the case for any of the texts examined in this section.

Another reason the poets and playwrights may have been incorporating yoga philosophy is to partake in the common phenomenon of *śāstrārtha*, as mentioned in section 1.9.[207] These debates occurred regularly in schools and royal courts. Any poet who received a formal education or who was embedded within the court through patronage or otherwise would have direct access to these ideas and displays of intellectual prowess. How could they not include

[206] Sheldon Pollock. "The Social Aesthetic and Sanskrit Literary Theory," *Journal of Indian Philosophy* 29, no. 1/2 (April 2021), 197-229: 198.
[207] Shiva Kumar Mishra, *Educational Ideas and Institutions in Ancient India: From the Earliest Times to 1206 A.D. With Special Reference to Mithilā* (New Delhi: Ramanand Vidya Bhawan, 1998), 3.

philosophy in their poems, whether by directly participating via these works or as an object of the poem?

Three of the four texts examined in this section were likely composed in the familiarity of courtly life. In addition, these writers received significant education that contributed to their ability to conceive of and portray philosophy in poetic ways. Mishra (1998) points out that in Kālidāsa's time, fourteen schools of thought were taught: "four Vedas and six Vedāṅgas, Mīmāṃsa, Nyāya, Purāṇa and Dharmaśāstra, Chanda, Mantra, Nirukta, Jyotiṣa, Grammar, Dhanurveda, Āyurveda and Gāndharvaveda."[208]

It is unlikely that every pupil was taught all of those schools, but at least in education hubs like Mithilā (in present-day Bihar), students were encouraged to go to various schools as they saw fit, so they had access to various streams of thought.[209] Importantly, Yoga and Sāṃkhya are not listed here, so while the poets had formal education in some philosophical schools, they did not appear to have education in the topics of analysis of this thesis. However, the broad philosophy education would have given them the tools necessary to better understand alternative philosophies. We see evidence of this in the *Prabodhacandrodaya*, which serves as an example of how important kāvya was within the world of philosophical debate. Despite being a satirical play, it is still considered one of the best commentaries on the philosophical schools of India.[210] Thus, I think it would be inaccurate to say that kāvya is not part of the ongoing debate between different schools of thought, and the fact that they included Yoga philosophy and practice tells us that they thought it was worth writing about—that it was a popular enough system of thought that it warranted attention.

208 Mishra, *Educational Ideas and Institutions in Ancient India*, 76.
209 Mishra, *Educational Ideas and Institutions in Ancient India*, 3.
210 Mishra, *Educational Ideas and Institutions in Ancient India*, 114.

I have two questions in mind for the analysis of these texts: Is there a difference between theory and practice of yoga? And can representations in kāvya help us understand practice? So far in this thesis, we have mostly examined theory and practice separately. In the first section, we looked exclusively at theory. In the second section, we looked at a mix of theory and practice, but rarely did the two overlap; either the texts were translations of theory, or they depicted the practices without explaining the theory. The Sanskrit texts I examine in this section are unique because their authors tend to include philosophy as well as practice in their descriptions. From the evidence, it appears that while kāvya poets were not yogis themselves, they had first-hand familiarity with yoga as an emergent system of philosophy and religious practice. The descriptions they provide are coherent and easily identifiable as yogis, especially when compared to the various yoga treatises detailed in section one. Their individual feelings about the philosophy or practices are not necessarily in line with each other, or in a positive light, but they—at least superficially—appear to be comfortable engaging with yoga topics and yogis with some sort of ease.

3.2 Kālidāsa's *Kumārasambhava* (300-400 CE)

The earliest work of Sanskrit kāvya I explore is called *Kumārasambhava* ("Birth of Kumāra") and was written by Kālidāsa in the fourth or fifth century CE. He lived in northern India, likely under the patronage of the Gupta dynasty. He was a devotee of Śiva.[211] Other than that, we do not know much about him. He was roughly contemporary with Patañjali so may have been aware of *Pātañjala Yogaśāstra*, though there are no direct quotes from the PYS in the *Kumārasambhava*—or any other work of Kālidāsa—that suggest he was. While some scholars,

[211] William J. Johnson, "Kālidāsa," *A Dictionary of Hinduism* (Oxford: Oxford University Press, 2009).

such as Kalia (2006), have suggested that portions of the KS are spurious, the descriptions of the *tapasyā* (ascetic practices) of Pārvatī and Śiva are generally thought to have been composed by Kālidāsa himself.[212] These extensive descriptions of ascetic practices give us an important artistic vision of yoga, though, as I argue below, Kālidāsa does not appear to be writing about yoga as in PYS, but about ascetic practices that predate formalized yoga schools. The value of these ascetic practices, for Kālidāsa, was ultimately in their potential as aesthetic imagery, and not to promote or teach a particular doctrine.

The *Kumārasambhava* is a poem that deals with the courtship and marriage of Śiva and Pārvatī, and the birth of their son Kumāra. This poem is a *mahākāvya*, a genre that typically deals with "political and military subjects" and is known for "a framework for long series of descriptions."[213] While the *Kumārasambhava* does fit this framework, it does not deal with political or military subjects but rather focuses on dramatic action, which is unusual for the genre. Tubb (1984) argues that Kālidāsa's decision to have the focus of the poem be on the heroine—Pārvatī—also displaces it from the genre of *mahākāvya*, as "Women appear in the definitions [of mahākāvya] only as recommended objects of description and as accessories in the sensual enjoyments included in the standard lists of topoi."[214] In theatre, however, theorists suggest that the heroine can be the subject in relation to the man she belongs to—normally the husband—or for her sexual experiences and appeal.[215] Certainly, Pārvatī, who is known for her unequaled beauty, fits that theme. The *rasa* most heavily involved in the *Kumārasambhava* is

---

[212] Ashok Kumar Kalia, "Forward," in *A Textual Study of Kumārasambhava* (Varanasi: Sampurnanand Sanskrit University, 2007), ii.
[213] Gary A. Tubb, "Heroine as Hero: Pārvatī in the Kumārasaṃbhava and the Pārvatīpariṇaya," *Journal of the American Oriental Society* 104, no. 2 (April-June 1984): 221.
[214] Tubb, "Heroine as Hero," 222; see also Gary A. Tubb, "Baking Umā," in *Innovations and Turning Points: Toward a History of Kāvya Literature*, edited by Yigal Bronner, David Shulman, and Gary Tubb (Oxford: Oxford University Press, 2014), 71-85.
[215] Tubb, "Heroine as Hero," 225-6.

that of *śṛṅgāra* (love or passion).[216] As part of Kālidāsa's explorations of śṛṅgāra, something fascinating happens in the fifth sarga, or canto. Pārvatī, upset that Śiva is not paying attention to her, curses her beauty and decides to practice extreme asceticism in the hope of gaining Śiva's appreciation. Since Śiva is known for being an accomplished yogi,[217] Pārvatī believes that the only way to gain his love is through practicing asceticism, since her extreme beauty did not interest him. That is to say, Kālidāsa imagines Pārvatī as becoming a *yoginī*, a female practitioner of yoga, in this poem, by description.

Asceticism does not necessarily mean being a yogi in the sense of a separate school, as we saw in section one. It was not until after Patañjali that yogis were considered a distinct school. However, the fact that Śiva is being so blatantly invoked as both a yogi and an object of affection is proof that this was not just a text about asceticism, but of asceticism *for the sake of* union with the divine—literally, in this case, through marriage and consummation. Union—in the sense of Puruṣa and Prakṛti, not marriage—is one of the earliest goals of yoga practice as a separate institution from other religions. The earliest representation of Śiva as existing outside the boundaries of society, as a disruptor and transgressor, is in the *Taittirīyasaṃhitā* (TS), which is embedded in the *Yajurveda* and composed roughly around the sixth century BCE.[218] In the TS, he is named Rudra, and had not yet taken the form of Śiva that he later became known as. He also appears as Rudra in the *Ṛg Veda* (10.136), wherein a "long-haired (*keśin*) sage or *muni*" is described as sharing a drug with him.[219] It is suggested in that text that he is a naked sage who controls his sexual power. Considering the *Kumārasambhava* depicts Śiva as an ascetic who is

---

[216] Tubb, "Heroine as Hero," 226.

[217] For instance, KS 3.50 describes Śiva as practicing what sounds very much like yoga as described in the PYS, with his mind controlled by deep concentration and looking upon the self within: *mano navadvāraniṣiddhavṛtti hṛdi vyavasthāpya samādhivaśyam | yam akṣaraṃ kṣetravido vidus tam ātmānam ātmany avalokayantam ||*

[218] Samuel, *The Origins of Yoga and Tantra*, 114.

[219] Samuel, *The Origins of Yoga and Tantra*, 158.

uninterested in sexual activity until Pārvatī also becomes a successful ascetic, it seems that Kālidāsa likely used these earlier forms as inspiration rather than the PYS or any other text belonging to the philosophical school of yoga, which makes sense given that the PYS was relatively contemporary to Kālidāsa's time so probably had not left as much of an impact yet. Indeed, it is not until the end of the Gupta period (c. 500 CE), that we see the full transformation to "theistic cult of deities, Śiva and Viṣṇu."[220] Śiva is also seen in relation to the *liṅga* as early as the Gupta dynasty, which can be both a formless and phallic representation of the god.[221] Since the *Kumārasambhava* also deals with the physical, consummatory union with Śiva, it seems safe to say Kālidāsa—and likely the society he was part of—were both familiar and comfortable with this proto-yogic depiction. It seems that Kālidāsa's poetry reflected the shifting perception of these deities—namely Rudra to Śiva—in the centuries leading up to the end of the dynasty. It is of course important to note that Patañjali did not include any name for Īśvara in the PYS, and seemed to suggest it was a formless, all-encompassing, transcendent deity. Thus, Kālidāsa's inclusion of Śiva's erotic aspect—and by extension a subtle reference to the liṅga representation—may be a sign that the formless, transcendental deity of PYS had not yet fully taken hold. However, in verse 5.78, Pārvatī does describe Śiva thus:

> [...] *na viśvamūrter avadhāryate vapuḥ* || 5.78 ||
>
> The body [of Śiva], whose form is the universe, is not known.

This is explicitly describing the formless, transcendental form of Śiva, so there is at least some admission by Kālidāsa that this is another aspect of the god, though it is not the primary one he is

---

[220] Samuel, *The Origins of Yoga and Tantra*, 195.

[221] Samuel, *The Origins of Yoga and Tantra*, 203. It is important to note that the liṅga form is not particularly popular until the fifth and sixth centuries CE, which is after Kālidāsa's time, though not long. It is possible that the forms of Śiva were established before the image of the liṅga was created.

concerned with. Whether or not the īśvara of PYS had taken hold, Kālidāsa was narrating a Purāṇic story about Śiva so it would be counter-productive to depict him as formless.[222]

Along with this relatively-early-influenced depiction of Śiva, Pārvatī's status as a yogi—and a very successful one at that—can tell us a few things about yogis in the fourth and fifth centuries, or at least of Kālidāsa's perception of them. Firstly, women were likely allowed to practice asceticism, but it was still secondary to their place as a romantic or sexual object in service of the men in their lives—at least in poetry. This does not mean, however, that women were expected to be ascetics, and how it is discussed in this play suggests that Pārvatī's actions were extraordinary. Secondly, there was not a widespread structured school of yoga so to speak, but rather Pārvatī is just described as a yogi because she performs ascetic practices. However, the suggestion of yogic practice that leads to union and includes practices done in a manner like that described in the PYS, and parallel to many Śaiva ascetic practices, does show the emergence of more structured yoga schools. While the PYS does not explicitly talk about union, it describes yoga as harnessing the mind for the purpose of samādhi, the state in which the yogi is entirely absorbed in puruṣa (spirit). Lastly, while Śiva is praised for performing extremely dedicated austerities, the focal point of the first half of the poem is that he is too focused on austerity for the sake of austerity and is forgoing his other duties; Pārvatī's practice on the other hand is geared towards achieving a particular goal rather than just for the sake of austerity itself and the prescriptive, individualized path to liberation described in the PYS.

As mentioned earlier, Pārvatī's practice was for the sake of union with Śiva, and a later chapter of the text deals explicitly with the consummation of their marriage. Even before that,

[222] Śaivism was emerging as an independent school of belief in the early medieval period and is found in epigraphy as early as the fourth century; see Alexis Sanderson, "The Śaiva Age: The Rise and Dominance of Śaivism During the Early Medieval Period," in *Genesis and Development of Tantrism*, edited by Shingo Einoo (Tokyo: Institute of Oriental Culture, University of Tokyo, 2009), 44.

Kālidāsa, when describing Pārvatī's ascetic practice, uses explicitly sexual descriptions of her. For example:

> *vimucya sā hāram ahāryaniścayā vilolayaṣṭipraviluptacandanam* |
> *babandha bālāruṇababhru valkalaṃ payodharotsedhaviśīrṇasaṃhati* || 5.8 ||
>
> In her immovable determination, she cast off her necklace whose swinging strings had already removed the sandalwood paste from her neck. She wore bark cloth that was the brown color of the early dawn and its stitches were pulled apart by the thickness of her breasts.

At the beginning of this section, I noted that the depiction of women in mahākāvya was often only for the sake of their sexual or aesthetic pleasures, but also that Kālidāsa was doing something different with this poem. It may be that he was adding these sexualized descriptions in because they were standard for this type of poetry, or it may be that he was mirroring the phallic liṅga aspect of Śiva in his depictions of her. In other words, Pārvatī is being sexualized in order to show that she has both the ascetic and sexualized aspects. For Śiva, in this text, asceticism comes first and sexualization comes second. For Pārvatī, sexualization comes first, then asceticism, then sexualization again. While at first this seems confusing—why treat the two differently while simultaneously showing they are the same?—it can be explained by what Pathak (2022) has called a "postpoststructuralist" interpretation of the "classical Śiva" period that ranged between circa 500 BCE and 500 CE.[223] Pathak argues that there are four eras of Śiva-progression. The earliest era was the structuralist Vedic Rudra (c. 1500-500 BCE), wherein Rudra/Śiva is one god with contradictory attributes, i.e. formed and formless, chaotic and peaceful. The second era was the classical era that Kālidāsa is writing in. The third era is the poststructuralist medieval Śiva (c. 500-1500 CE) wherein the oppositional aspects require Śiva to

[223] Pathak, "Shifting Śāstric Śiva: Co-operating Epic Mythology and Philosophy in India's Classical Period," *International Journal of Hindu Studies* 27, 2022.

split into the masculine and feminine form of Śiva-Pārvatī to accommodate the contradictions. The fourth era is the modern Śiva (c. 1500 CE to present) where the poststructuralist separation of one into two remains. In examining the classical era, Pathak utilizes a postpoststructuralist perspective that claims all the options were included by Kālidāsa because he was giving voice to all interpretations of Śiva that existed in society at the time. That is, society's view of Śiva was shifting between the conception of him as one god that included all attributes and a god that had to split into different forms in order for the aspects to operate. Kālidāsa skillfully included both options by describing Śiva as formless while having form and having him reunite with Pārvatī as his other half. Indeed, the narrative of Pārvatī being reborn after the Sati incarnation so that she can remarry Śiva is indicative of the cycle of separation and union between the two opposing forces—though not without significant effort on Pārvatī's part.

Here is a list of the actual practices Pārvatī undertook in the *Kumārasambhava* in her attempt to woo Śiva: went to a mountain (5.7), wore bark for clothing (5.8), had matted hair (5.9), wore a *maunja* cord (5.10), had a rosary (5.11), slept on the bare ground (5.12), ritually bathed, offered fire oblations, and recited sacred texts (5.16), sat amongst four fires in the heat of summer (5.20),[224] severely fasted (5.22), and stood in cold water while it snowed (5.26). These are all ascetic practices, but not specifically yogic practices. Many of them are included in PYS, but they also appear in the Vedas and earlier texts separately from the philosophical school of yoga. There is nothing in these descriptions of Pārvatī that suggest she was practicing *yoga*.

Ultimately, the religio-philosophical landscape was shifting in Kālidāsa's time and that is reflected in this text with the inclusion of both physical descriptions of Śiva and identifying him

[224] This practice of sitting in between four fires and staring at the sun is still commonly practiced by Hindu ascetics. The analogy is of course a connection to the five sacred Vedic fires, as per Patrick Olivelle, "The Early History of Renunciation," in *The Oxford History of Hinduism*, edited by Gavin Flood (Oxford: Oxford Univeristy Press, 2020) 102.

as formless, in the practices Pārvatī undertakes, and in the ultimate goal of literal union between Śiva and Pārvatī. While this text does not appear to be inspired by a formalized yoga school, the seeds of what is included—and expanded upon—in the PYS are there. Placing the KS as the first of our analysis of yoga in Sanskrit kāvya literature is an important baseline against which the other texts can be compared. Are they giving the same descriptions or different ones? Is there more direct evidence of yoga specifically? How has the perception of Śiva changed? I will try to answer these questions in the following sections.

3.3 Māgha's *Śiśupālavadha* (600-700 CE)

The second kāvya to be examined is the *Śiśupālavadha* ("Slaying of Śiśuplāla"), which was written by Māgha, who lived around the seventh to eighth century of the Common Era. Like Kālidāsa, not much is known about Māgha. He says nothing about himself in his text, and since only the *Śiśupālavadha* (SV) is attributed to him, very little can be gleaned regarding his identity. While we do not know much about him, Māgha takes a very intellectual approach to yoga in his texts, not just by including verses specifically from Yoga and Sāṃkhya philosophies but also in his imagery and underlying suggestions.

Like the *Kumārasambhava*, the *Śiśupālavadha* is a mahākāvya. It consists of 20 sargas that are inspired by the story of Kṛṣṇa slaying his cousin Śiśupāla in the *Mahābharata*. In summary, Kṛṣṇa is invited to a *rājasuya* ceremony (consecration of the king) for Yudhiṣṭhira. The story includes a few scenes, including his journey to the city where the ceremony is held, the ceremony itself, and an honor bestowed upon Kṛṣṇa to which Śiśupāla gets angered and causes a scene. The two end up at war against each other, and at the end, Kṛṣṇa cuts off Śiśupāla's head.

The SV is relevant to this thesis because it includes quotations and paraphrases directly from Sāṃkhya and Yoga texts, as noted by Chatterjee and Mondal (2014), and Freschi and Maas (2017). In addition, Bronner and McCrea (2012) and Salomon (2014) have shown that there are two alternative readings in passages 14.14-39; the original reading, as argued by them, is critical of Kṛṣṇa. If their analysis is correct, then it may be that Māgha was interested in venerating Śiva, despite the text centering around Kṛṣṇa; this theory is supported by Māgha's inclusion of various yoga philosophies and even stating in 14.61 that Kṛṣṇa actually encompasses all three major deities, one of which is of course Śiva. However, Maas (2017) provides an alternative interpretation in that by placing Kṛṣṇa as the "capstone" of the trinity, so to speak, Māgha is effectively identifying Kṛṣṇa as "the unnamed transcendental God of classical Yoga theology."[225] Maas gives the other example of stanza 14.60, where yogis are defined "as a group of devotees to Viṣṇu-Kṛṣṇa, for whom God is the object of their meditation," to support this reading.[226] It seems more likely that Māgha was neither a Vaiṣṇavite nor a Śaivite, but rather a hybrid, or perhaps he considered God as indeed just the unnamed transcendental God in yoga theology and only named it as anything in particular to appeal to his readers.

Identifying the author's personal beliefs with any amount of certainty may not be possible, but we can glean what knowledge the author had, and indeed how he approached yoga, by looking at the text. Which verses of the SV specifically are thought to be from Sāṃkhya and Yoga texts? Verses 1.31-33, 4.55, 13.23, and 14.62. An examination of each verse is below.

[225] Philipp A. Maas, "From Theory to Poetry: The Reuse of Patañjali's Yogaśāstra in Māgha's Śiśupālavadha," in *Adaptive Reuse*, edited by Elisa Freschi and Philipp A. Maas, 29-62 (Germany: Deutsche Morgenländische Gesellschaft, 2017), 50.
[226] Maas, "From Theory to Poetry," 50.

iti bruvantam tam uvāca sa vratī
na vācyam ittham puruṣottama tvayī |
tvam eva sākṣātkaraṇīya ity ataḥ
kim asti kāryam guru yogināṃ api || 1.31 ||

The ascetic said to [Lord Kṛṣṇa] who had spoken: Oh, greatest of men! This should not be said by you, since you are the one who is manifested. Therefore, what other action is greater than this for yogis?

udīrṇarāgapratirodhakaṃ janair
abhīkṣṇam akṣuṇṇatayātidurgamam |
upeyuṣo mokṣapathaṃ manasvinas
tvam agrabhūmir nirapāyasaṃśrayā || 1.32 ||

For the wise man who is traveling on a path of liberation that is very difficult to traverse by people who are inexperienced, is the thing that obstructs excited passion, you are the high land.

udāsitāraṃ nigṛhītamānasair
gṛhītam adhyātmadṛśā kathaṃcana |
bahirvikāraṃ prakṛteḥ pṛthag viduḥ
purātanaṃ tvāṃ puruṣaṃ purāvidaḥ || 1.33 ||

The knowers of the past, seeing with their inner self, knew you to be the ancient/primordial, indifferent puruṣa who is outside of change and who is separate from prakṛti (matter), who is grasped by those whose mind is restrained/controlled.

These three verses are not direct quotations from a text, but they describe the nature of the world through a Sāṃkhya philosophical lens. As we saw in the first section, this school of philosophy considers puruṣa and prakṛti to be separate (reflected in SV 1.31 and 1.33), is accepting of an inner self (SV 1.33), and teaches that we should learn to control our mind in order to become liberated and understand these truths (SV 1.32 and 1.33).

**

maitryādicittaparikarmavido vidhāya
kleśaprahāṇam iha labdhasabījayogāḥ |
khyātiṃ ca sattvapuruṣānyatayādhigamya
vāñchanti tām api samādhibhṛto nirodhum || 4.55 ||

> Wise men, knowing the preparation of the mind with care etc., abandon the afflictions and here obtain conceptual yogic meditations. Having discovered the difference of pure awareness and subtle cognition, the renowned practitioners of absorption wish even to transcend that.

This verse is talking explicitly about yoga practice. If you did not know it was part of a poem, you might think it was part of a yoga text. Indeed, Maas (2017) identifies this verse as a reuse of PYS 1.32-3,[227] in which the path to liberation is described. This verse shows up in the section of the poem where Dāruka, Kṛṣṇa's charioteer, is describing the mountain Raivataka to him. The section begins by an un-narrated description of the beauty of the mountain before Dāruka steps in to elaborate on it. It is in Dāruka's narration that we see verse 4.55. It is not just the fact that this specific verse is a quotation of the PYS, but the fact that it comes within a section narrated by the charioteer is reminiscent of an ongoing motif in South Asian literature, the Chariot Analogy (*Ratha Kalpana*).[228] This motif has its origin in chapter three of the *Kaṭha Upaniṣad* (KU):

> *ātmānaṃ rathinaṃ viddhi śarīraṃ ratham eva tu* |
> *buddhiṃ tu sārathiṃ viddhi manaḥ pragraham eva ca* || 3.3 ||
> *indriyāṇi hayān āhur viṣayāṃs teṣu gocarān* |
> *ātmendriyamanoyuktaṃ bhoktety āhur manīṣiṇaḥ* ||3.4 ||

> "3.3 Know the self as a rider in a chariot,
> and the body, as simply the chariot.
> Know the intellect as the charioteer,
> and the mind, as simply the reins.
> 3.4. The senses, they say, are the horses,
> and sense objects are the paths around them;
> He who is linked to the body (ātman), senses, and mind,
> the wise proclaim as the one who enjoys."[229]

---

227 Maas, "From Theory to Poetry," 38.
228 Allan Jones, *Beyond Vision: Going Blind, Inner Seeing, and the Nature of the Self* (Canada: McGill-Queen's University Press, 2018), 89.
229 Patrick Olivelle, ed. and trans., *Upaniṣads* (Oxford: Oxford University Press, 1996), 238-9.

The KU is not a text about yoga; indeed, it came long before yoga was a defined school of practice and philosophy. But some scholars, like Larson (1969), have posited that this section marks the beginnings of Sāṃkhya thought,[230] which we have already established in section one forms the basis of yogic philosophy also.

The next place we see this motif is the *Bhagavad Gītā* (BG), with Kṛṣṇa as Arjuna's charioteer. This depiction is important to our cause as it is the first time where the charioteer is represented as a separate individual (specifically a transcendental divine being) who provides knowledge to the rider—specifically knowledge about yoga. Now, we see Māgha evoking this same motif in this section in which he includes an explicit yoga teaching by Dāruka to—ironically—Kṛṣṇa about how to reach enlightenment. Subjugating Kṛṣṇa to the position of learning from the charioteer seems to suggest that Māgha believes he is not the transcendental divine being. This might be a metaphor for the teachings of yoga evolving beyond what Kṛṣṇa taught to Arjuna in the BG, but on the surface, it reads like Māgha is almost mocking Kṛṣṇa's knowledge, or at least playing with irony that would be appreciated by learned audiences.

The physical environment utilized in this context is important to note. Specifically, Dāruka states that a mountain is the best place to practice yoga, which reflects the general sentiment of ascetics and yogis across time, as well as what we saw in the KS.[231] Various primary yoga texts detail suitable places to practice yoga and meditation, and most are desolate, free from distractions, and close to nature. An example is in the HYP (1.12-4) where the best place for a yogi to practice is described in specific detail, even down to the size of the room.[232]

---

[230] Gerald James Larson, *Classical Sāṃkhya: An Interpretation of its History and Meaning* (Delhi: Motilal Banarsidas Publishers Private Ltd., 1969), 97.
[231] Maas, "From Theory to Poetry," 45.
[232] While the HYP obviously comes later than the SV, the idea is as old as the *Upaniṣads* wherein the tales describe ascetics living in forests and other remote regions such as mountains.

There is no way having the yoga teachings in a section with a charioteer and the mountains is a coincidence, and it only adds evidence that Māgha was intentionally embedding yoga teachings in the poem—explicitly and subtly.

> **
> *vaśinaṃ kṣiter ayanayāviveśvaraṃ*
> *niyamo yamaś ca niyataṃ yatiṃ yathā* |
> *vijayaśriyā vṛtam ivārkamārutā-*
> *vanusasratustamatha dasrayoḥ sutau* || 13.23 ||
>
> Iśvara (lord of the earth) is followed by fortune and virtue, just like earth is followed by the sun and the wind, Yati (an ascetic) is followed by Yama and Niyama, Kṛṣṇa is followed by the two sons (of Mādarī, Nakula and Sahadeva).

The interesting part about this verse is the second line in which yamas and niyamas are said to "follow" the ascetic. As a reminder these are the moral principles and observances that yogis are supposed to adhere to as early as the PYS. This shows that not only was Patañjali's yoga practiced, but it was also in the forefront of Māgha's mind. In Vallabhadeva's tenth-century commentary of this verse,[233] the following yamas and niyamas are listed:

> *ahiṃsā satyāsteya brahmacaryā-parigrahā yamāḥ* |
> *śauca-santoṣa-svādhyāye-śvarapraṇidhānāni niyamāḥ* ||
>
> It is said: the moral principles are nonviolence, truthfulness, non-stealing, celibacy, and generosity. The observances are cleanliness, contentment, study, and devotion to God.

This list is almost the same as that found in PYS, only leaving out *tapas* (austerity) from the *niyamas*, which speaks more to the commentator's knowledge or preference than the verse itself, or perhaps that the list had changed during the few hundred years between PYS and Vallabhadeva. Alternatively, it may have been that the list was borrowing from a different tradition that placed tapas in the yamas or excluded it altogether, as we saw in the *Yoga*

[233] Vallabhadeva quotes the *Yoga Darśana* 2.31, which was the original commentary on the PYS and is thought to be the same author, as shown in the first section, according to Maas (2013).

Yajñavalkya. As I detailed in the first section, the contents of the yamas and niyamas did not remain consistent throughout all yoga texts or schools.

> **
> *sarva vedinam anādim āsthitaṃ*
> *dehinām anujighṛkṣayā vapuḥ* |
> *kleśa karma phala bhogavarjitaṃ*
> *puṃviśeṣam amum īśvaraṃ viduḥ* || 14.62 ||
>
> He who knows all, without beginning, obtained a body with the desire to give favour to embodied beings. Devoid of the fruits of karma and the afflictions, this God [is] a special kind of consciousness.

Lastly, 14.62 is the final verse that brings in PYS. This comes at the beginning of a speech by Bhīṣma that introduces Kṛṣṇa as the guest of honor. This is the section wherein Bronner and McCrea (2012) and Salomon (2014) identify Māgha's original version as being critical of Kṛṣṇa. Their argument is based on the fact that the speech given in response to Bhīṣma by Śiśupāla denounces Kṛṣṇa, accusing him of not being an incarnation of Viṣṇu. This scene is in the second book of the *Mahābhārata* (2.33-42). In Māgha's version, however, Śiśupāla's speech is drawn out and Bronner and McCrea (2012) and Salomon (2014) all agree that this long version of the speech was meant to be accusatory towards Kṛṣṇa's character, rather than an alternative reading that could be taken as either blame or praise. I am inclined to agree with their reading given that, earlier in the poem, Kṛṣṇa was depicted as requiring yoga teachings, as noted in verse 4.55.

In this verse's description of the aspects of God, it reuses PYS 1.24-5, stanzas that also describe Īśvara as unaffected by afflictions and karma.[234] This is a divergence from the complementary features of the divine that Kālidāsa balanced in his earlier text and suggests that

---

[234] Maas, "From Theory to Poetry," 47.

Māgha and his audience were comfortable with a transcendental deity as posited in yoga philosophy, and as opposed to earlier iteration.

Even though this text is dealing with Kṛṣṇa and not Śiva, it is clearly dealing with yoga concepts and promoting the practices in such a way as to suggest that Māgha was actually critical of Kṛṣṇa, was familiar with PYS and Sāṃkhya philosophies, and was willing to let go of the older forms of theology to adopt the newer forms. Another framing of this is that Māgha was not critical of Kṛṣṇa himself, but of the yoga as described in the *Bhagavad Gītā,* and is instead focused on promoting the yoga from PYS. Since yogis themselves are not depicted in this text, it is not possible to assess whether people were actually practicing the yoga and Sāṃkhya teachings, or if Māgha was just sympathetic towards them. However, given that the SV was composed a couple hundred years after the PYS, it is likely that people were practicing the PYS as it was taught for it to be worthy of inclusion in this epic poem.

3.4 Kṛṣṇamiśra's *Prabodhacandrodaya* (1100 CE)

The *Prabodhacandrodaya*, ("The Rise of the Wisdom Moon") was composed sometime between 1042 and 1098 of the Common Era. Kṛṣṇamiśra, the author, was a Vaiṣnava and Vedāntin, which influenced the way he portrayed the characters in this play, as we will see in some of his specific statements about them. I mentioned in the introduction to this section that one of the reasons poems might include philosophy is as a method of teaching. Here, we might see an example of that. It is speculated that Kṛṣṇamiśra was an ascetic in the Haṃsa order of the Advaita school and wrote the play to teach the Advaita doctrine to his disciples.[235]

---

[235] Sita Krishna Nambiar, *Prabodhacandrodaya of Kṛṣṇa Miśra: Sanskrit Text with English Translation, A Critical Introduction and Index* (Delhi: Motilal Banarsidass, 1971), 1-2.

The *Prabodhacandrodaya* (PC) begins after a battle wherein a lord named Gopāla helped King Kīrtivarman win the throne. After they celebrate, Gopāla wants to encourage spiritual peace and so has a play that was written by his guru, Kṛṣṇamiśra, performed in front of King Kīrtivarman, that will teach how to overcome ignorance. The PC takes place in this meta-narrative. Each of the characters are named after a quality of mind or a religious figure, such as Kāma (Lust), Śānti (Peace), Māna (Pride) and Dambha (Deceit). Most important for our cause is Act 3, where Śānti is in search of her mother, Śraddhā (Faith). As she travels about to find her, she comes across various other figures who claim to be her mother but are ultimately proven not to be as they expound their philosophies and are deemed inadequate. Those figures are Digambara/ Kṣapaṇaka (Jain), Bhikṣu (Buddhist), and Somasiddhānta/ Kāpālika (Śaivite/ "Skullman"). The allegory here is that these three religions are not true faiths.

Utilizing satire, Kṛṣṇamiśra subordinated Śaivism, Buddhism, and Jainism to the Vedānta teachings he was promoting, and further subordinated Yoga by not acknowledging it as its own school, but rather as "a method that aids one on the path to liberation."[236] As Sathaye (2022) notes, satire provides the audience with the ability to view fringe religious figures from afar, without fear of being implicated for it.[237] Unusually, in Act 5, the teachings of Vaiṣṇava, Śaiva, and others are brought under the umbrella of Vedānta philosophy in an inclusive way, on the "good side" of the battle against the negative states of being, such as Kāma, Māna, and Dambha.[238] While ultimately the Buddhist, Jains, and Śaivites fight on the "good" Vedānta side,

---

[236] Michael S. Allen, "Dueling Dramas, Dueling Doxographies: The Prabodhacandrodaya and Saṃkalpasūryodaya," *The Journal of Hindu* Studies 9 (2016): 276.
[237] Adheesh Sathaye, "How the Guru Lost His Power: Public Anxieties of Tantric Knowledge in the Sanskrit *Vetāla* Tales," in *Religious Authority in South Asia*, edited by István Keul and Srilata Raman (London: Routledge, 2022), 10.
[238] Allen, "Dueling Dramas, Dueling Doxograhpies," 278.

they end up leaving after the fight to live amongst the Huns, outcastes and non-Vedāntic faiths (5.44), so it is not a complete acceptance but still better than being outright discarded.

Later in this section, I will examine how Śraddha (Faith) is portrayed, which leads me to the conclusion, along with the above-mentioned inclusivity and subjugation, that Kṛṣṇamiśra thought Jainism, Buddhism, and Śaivism were wrong faiths, but that they were still close enough to the Vedās and Vedānta to be considered in some kind of harmony (5.38).[239] While that may seem strange considering these religions deny the validity of the Veda, it appears to be the position Kṛṣṇamiśra promoted. Yoga, on the other hand, is not acknowledged by Kṛṣṇamiśra as a separate faith, and I will examine why that might be below.

One of the things we might consider for the purposes of this analysis is the inclusion of not just Sanskrit in this play but also Prakrit. In a later play written in response to the PC, *Saṃkalpasūryodaya* by Vedāntadeśika, c. 1370 CE,[240] there is a quote that speaks to the purpose of this linguistic switch: "the Buddhists, Jainas and others are to be laughed at because they compose their canonical works in various Prakrit dialects."[241] Prakrit was used in plays as early as Bhāsa, the first known dramatist from the third century CE, and the specific language usage changed over time as the language itself evolved. Regardless, its use indicated someone was uneducated in Sanskrit. While some scholars, such as Warder (2011), think the use of Prakrit is meant to show someone was generally irreligious and uneducated, thus subjugating them to Sanskrit speakers, other scholars like Ollett (2017) and Pollock (2006) claim Prakrit was a literary language with at least as much textual production as that in Sanskrit. Of the three

---

[239] *samānānvayajātānāṃ parasparavirodhinām | paraiḥ pratyabhibhūtānāṃ prasūte saṅgatiḥ śriyam ||*

[240] The *Saṃkalpasūryodaya* includes the same characters, other than Ego and Mind, which were left out entirely. Vedāntadeśika added Saṃkalpa (Intention), Abhiniveśa (Addiction), Kuhanā (Hypocrisy), and Saṃskāra (Artist). While Kṛṣṇamiśra's play was allegorical, this "remix" has been described as aesthetically bland: "the calmed śānta is the only real aesthetic experience: the rest just cancel each other out," as per Anthony Kennedy Warder, *Indian Kāvya Literature, Volume VIII: The Performance of Kāvya in the +14* (Delhi: Motilal Banarsidass, 2011), 302.

[241] Warder, *Indian Kāvya Literature, Volume VIII*, 305.

religious figures in this part of the text, it is only the Jain that speaks in Prakrit; the Buddhist and Śaivite both speak in Sanskrit. However, it was Jains that are known for producing their texts in Prakrit, while Buddhists utilized whatever language was local to the practicing population.[242] According to Ollett (2017), it is generally recognized that Prakrit was "first employed as a textual language" in commentaries on Jain canonical literature, and the fact that Kṛṣṇamiśra chose to use Prakrit only for the Jain likely serves as evidence supporting that.[243] Thus, the use of Prakrit in the PC by the Jain may well only be due to the use of it in Jain literary production, and any comical undertones may only be being read into the performance by the audience, since it is not stated explicitly in the text itself.

The character we are interested in is that of the Somasiddhānta (Śaivite), who is called *Kāpālika* (skull-bearer) when people realize what he practices. Importantly, while tantric practitioners are sometimes referred to as Kāpālikas, this title does not necessarily indicate any particular sectarian order, nor is there any proof in texts, inscriptions, or otherwise that the practitioners would call themselves Kāpālikas.[244] It is important to note that Śiva is also known as Kapālin (see verse 5.71), also "Skull-bearer," so the term Kāpālika may be broadly indicative of people who follow Śiva's yogi form. Supporting this reading, non-Śaivites tended to use the term to indicate that the Śaiva ascetic orders were transgressive.[245] So it seems the use of this term in this play is likely derogatory. Very little is known about Kāpālikas, but it does seem apparent that the description of them given in the PC is equivalent to other sources, and so it can

---

[242] Andrew Ollett, *Language of the Snakes: Prakrit, Sanskrit, and the Language Order of Premodern India* (Oakland: University of California Press, 2017), 9.
[243] Ollett, *Language of the Snakes*, 9.
[244] David Gordon White, "Review of *Indian Esoteric Buddhism*, by R.M. Davidson," *Journal of the International Association of Tibetan Studies* 1: 1-11, 2005, 9.
[245] David N. Lorenzen, *The Kāpālikas and Kālāmukhas: Two Lost Śaivite Sects* (New Delhi: Thomson Press, 1972).

be assumed that Kṛṣṇamiśra was accurately aware of their beliefs and practices, or at least was invoking public tropes.[246]

The first introduction we have to this character is a verse that he is reciting:

> *narāsthimālākṛtacārubhūṣaṇaḥ*
> *smaśānavāsī nṛkapālabhojanaḥ* |
> *paśyāmi yogāñjanaśuddhacakṣuṣā*
> *jagan mitho bhinnam abhinnam īśvarāt* || 12 ||
>
> I wear attractive ornaments made of garlands of human bones, I am living in the cremation ground, and I eat my food out of a skull; I see, with eyes purified by yoga's balm, the world as being alternatively different from and not different from the Lord (Śiva).

While on the surface this is clearly a nondual philosophy, and this Śaivite is identifiably a tantric practitioner, the term *mithas* (mutually, alternatively) could suggest that Kṛṣṇamiśra was pointing out a hypocrisy in that the belief could be both dual and nondual. This may be because yoga was traditionally a dualistic philosophy until around the time of the *Amṛtasiddhi*, from which point, various schools became nondualist, as seen in the first section of this thesis. Keeping in mind that the *Amṛtasiddhi* was composed around the same time as the PC, it is likely that Kṛṣṇamiśra was lampooning the kinds of Nāth yoga traditions that were proliferating in the world around him.[247] In fact, "Tantrism" as an institution was transitioning from *tapas* (austerity) being the focus to

[246] Lorenzen, *The Kāpālikas and Kālāmukhas*. In his text, Lorenzen states a particular vow known as the Mahāvrata is what distinguishes the Kāpālikas from other tantric sects. The rules for performing this vow include the description of using a skull from a brahmin whom one accidentally killed as a drinking vessel (75). While this play does not suggest the Kāpālika killed a brahmin, it does depict him as using a skull as a cup.

[247] This is not to say that the *Amṛtasiddhi* was not doing something new, it of course was combining Vājrayāna Buddhist teachings with other tantric ideas, such as the Nāths. The fact that the text was written shows that the ideas were prevalent, even if they had not been written down by other traditions yet. This is also why analyzing literature is one way to determine what was being practiced—sometimes the poets and playwrights wrote about things they saw before the practices were textualized by the practitioners.

śakti (power), which is quite obviously the case in these descriptions.[248] He goes on to describe further practices:

> *mastiṣkāntravasābhipūritamahāmāṃsāhutīr juhvatāṃ*
> *vahnau brahmakapālakalpitasurāpānena naḥ pāraṇā* |
> *sadyaḥkṛttakaṭhorakaṇṭhavigalatkīlāladhārojjvalair*
> *arcyo naḥ puruṣopahārabalibhir devo mahābhairavaḥ* || 13 ||
>
> As we make the offering of human flesh, including brains, guts, and marrow (*vasā*), into the fire, it gets completed (*pāraṇa*) by our drinking liquor prepared in a brahmin's skull; our great lord Bhairava must be worshipped with sacrificial offerings of a human victim, blazing up with streams of blood oozing from its freshly cut thick neck.

He goes on to share not only beliefs, but also abilities he has been able to achieve through his practice:

> *(sakrodham) āḥ pāpa pākhaṇḍāpasada muṇḍitamuṇḍa cūḍālakeśa keśaluñcaka*
> *are vipralambhakaḥ kila caturdaśabhuvanotpattisthitipralayapravartako*
> *vedāntaprasiddhasiddhāntavibhavo bhagavān bhavānīpatiḥ* | *darśayāmas tarhi*
> *dharmasyāsya mahimānam* |
>
> (*With anger*) Oh you wicked, heretical outcast with a shaven head, who has a tuft of hair, and who pulls their hair out. Hey, this deceptive fellow is in fact Lord Śiva himself, husband of Bhavānī, who is the creator, sustainer, and destroyer of the fourteen worlds, and whose majesty comes from the well-established doctrines of the Vedānta. Let me now show you the greatness of this religion!
>
> *hariharasurajyeṣṭhaśreṣṭhān surān aham āhare*
> *viyati vahatāṃ nakṣatrāṇāṃ ruṇadhmi gatīr api* |
> *sanaganagarīmambhaḥpūrṇāṃ vidhāya mahīm imāṃ*
> *kalaya sakalaṃ bhūyas toyaṃ kṣaṇena pibāmi tat* || 14 ||
>
> I can deliver Hari, Hara, and the eldest and best of the gods. I can even obstruct the movement of constellations and stars which are situated in the sky; I can flood this earth with water, with its mountains and towns and— think of this!— drink up all that water again in a moment.

When asked specifically about the *saukhyamokṣa* (blissful freedom) that is the Skullbearer's "highest teaching," he responds:

---

[248] Po-chi Huang, "The Cult of Vetāla and Tantric Fantasy," in *Rethinking Ghosts in World Religions* (Numen Book Series, 2009), 211.

dṛṣṭaṃ kvāpi sukhaṃ vinā na viṣayair ānandabodhojjhitā
jīvasya sthitir eva muktir upalāvasthā kathaṃ prārthyate |
pārvatyāḥ pratirūpayā dayitayā sānandam āliṅgito
muktaḥ krīḍati candracūḍavapur ity ūce mṛḍānīpatiḥ || 16 ||

> Happiness is nowhere seen without materialities; so the living condition, though lacking awareness of bliss, is already liberation— how come it's described as a rock-like state? And so Śiva, the husband of lovely Pārvatī, had said that the Moon-crested Śiva is liberated as he joyously embraces and frolics with his beloved who is a counterfeit image of Pārvatī.

Śiva and Pārvatī are mentioned here, which on the surface seems unexceptional coming from a Śaivite. However, the suggestion of Śiva being interested in Pārvatī's *pratirūpā* (image, guise) is curious as it suggests the goddess is not present. Why would Śiva need to amuse himself with her image, rather than her real form? If Kṛṣnamiśra is using this text as a teaching tool for his students, this verse can be taken as describing the philosophical beliefs of the Kāpālika. If that is the case, it could be playing on the idea of *jīvanmukti* (*jīvasya sthitir eva muktiḥ*), which claims that liberation is already a condition of the living, so Śiva can be both liberated while also playing with a material image of the (equally liberated) Umā. If we dive deeper, it suggests that they are actually one form, and since it is impossible to see oneself, they can only experience likenesses of each other. Although, this does not necessarily follow the general idea of the splitting of the *ardhanārīśvara* form, in which they are combined and can separate to perform actions that require one end of the extreme, as mentioned in the *Kumārasambhava* section above. However, if Kṛṣṇamiśra is writing this text as satire, or trying to ridicule these groups, this description would suggest he is making fun of Śiva in such that he is so absorbed in sense objects that even he is unable to see the difference between the true goddess and her likeness.

As the scene progresses, each of the religious figures calls in Śraddhā (Faith) and she comes disguised as whatever suits the particular religion. For instance, when the Kāpālika calls her in, she comes as Kāpālinī, a female Kāpālika.[249] We find out in the beginning of Act 4 that she did not choose to appear when the non-Vedic religious figures called on her, but was forced to materialize. This suggests that Kṛṣṇamiśra acknowledges that each of these religions believe they are truly faithful, but really, they are just forcing faith to appear where it is not really present, or at least not as genuine faith. In other words, Śraddhā did not want to be a Kāpālinī, but she had to appear as such because the Kāpālika truly believed he was being faithful to the religion.

Now, Kāpālikas, while being tantric ascetics, are not necessarily yogis in the sense that they do not seem to consider themselves—at least in the context of this text—as anything other than Śaivites.[250] Importantly, the final goal of yoga was liberation—though what that looks like specifically depends on the school of yoga one practices—and so the fact that the Kāpālika is speaking directly against liberation and wants to promote the sensual pleasures shows that indeed he is not a yogi as the PYS school of thought would allow. Śaiva yoga sects may have been okay with the pursuit of worldly pleasure, at least in some capacity, but ultimately the goal of yoga as its own school of thought is liberation. There are of course similarities between Śaivites and yoga schools that were prevalent around the turn of the first millennium in that they are ascetics, tend to support Śiva (though to varying degrees), and practice some kind of meditation. There are also known Śaiva yoga sects. However, at least in the description of this text, the Kāpālikas do not practice for the same goal as yogis, and as noted earlier, practitioners are more interested in power in this period than asceticism.[251]

---

[249] *tataḥ praviśati kāpālinīrūpadhāriṇī śraddhā* || 3.101 ||

[250] At this point it is not possible to say how Kāpālikas considered themselves outside how other people depicted them because we have no known texts attributed to them, and as far as we know, they no longer exist in practice. See David N. Lorenzen, "Śaivism: Kāpālikas," in *Encyclopedia of Religion volume 12*, second edition (Detroit, MI: Macmillan Reference USA, 2005), *Gale E-Books*.

[251] This shift symbolizes a cognitive shift away from yoga as needing to control the senses, as in PYS, to being more interested in the body, as we see in the *Amṛtasiddhi*, where bodily practices such as postures, breathwork and

As we saw in verse twelve above, the Kāpālika does admit to practicing yoga in order to see the world clearly: "*paśyāmi yogāñjanaśuddhacakṣuṣā*" ("I see, with eyes purified by yoga's balm"). So, yoga is recognized as a tool with which one can acquire understanding and knowledge of the true nature of the world—whatever that true nature might be to the practitioner. We saw in the previous two texts that yoga was given substantial description, though in different ways. Kālidāsa was dealing with yoga as its pre-PYS form as strictly ascetic practice, which could be considered closer to the depiction of the practice of yoga found in the PC, however sparse. Māgha was very much interested in institutionalized yoga as found in the PYS and Sāṃkhya philosophy. It seems that, a few hundred years later, Kṛṣṇamiśra may be showing that institutionalized yoga was fractured and the perception had returned to being more about asceticism than a formal school of belief and practice. This could make sense, as the tradition that built upon the PYS was branching off into various other schools of yoga that were similar, yet different, as we saw in section one (and many more schools than we examined earlier). It could also show that Śaiva and Tantric features that were part of some of the newly developing yoga schools were part of the public understanding of yogic practice.

The depiction of Śiva in this text is much more in line with the medieval depiction as described by Pathak (2022) where Śiva and Pārvatī are two aspects of the same deity that must separate to perform action because when they are one, they basically cancel each other out with their opposing aspects. This is different than in the works of Kālidāsa and Māgha, which makes sense given the dates (the PC being composed in the eleventh century while the other two were composed in the middle of the first millennium). Ultimately, what we see in the PC is what we

energetic manipulation are prescribed. The depiction in the PC of these tantrics and yogis as being more interested in power than liberation is indicative of this shift being well-known by the contemporary populace, not just contained to the sects themselves.

would expect to see given the time the text was written. It does not seem to be providing any new depictions of yoga, yogis, or tantrics, that we would not find in other texts. What it is doing new is providing some sort of inclusion of the various religions that can acceptably—according to Kṛṣṇamiśra—fall under the umbrella of the Vedas, as shown in Act Five where the Buddhist, Jain and Śaivite are accepted under the banner of the Vedānta philosophy to fight on their side of the battle.

3.5 Vetālapañcaviṃśati (1000-1500 CE)

The *Vetālapañcavimśati* ("Twenty-Five Tales of the Animated Corpse") (VP) is a collection of tales about a king who promises a tantric guru that he will capture a vetāla, a spirit who takes possession of corpses,[252] and bring it to him. The earliest extant version of these tales was in the eleventh century by a Sanskrit polymath from Kashmir named Kṣemendra, and shortly thereafter by Somadeva, and there have been many iterations and translations into various languages since.[253] There are four major Sanskrit "tellings"—to borrow A.K. Ramanujan's term—[254]of the tales that have survived to the present day, and my analysis is mostly taken from Śivadāsa's version as edited and translated by Sathaye (Forthcoming).[255] Śivadāsa's version of the tales were written for the amusement and education of a Sanskrit-educated public audience,

[252] W. J. Johnson, "Vetāla," in *A Dictionary of Hinduism* (Oxford: Oxford University Press, 2009).
[253] David Adams Leeming, *Storytelling Encyclopedia: Historical, Cultural, and Multiethnic Approaches to Oral Traditions Around the World.* (Arizona: Oryx Press, 1997), 337.
[254] Attipat Krishnaswami Ramanujan, "Three Hundred Rāmāyaṇas: Five Examples and Three Thoughts on Translation," in *The Collected Essays of A.K. Ramanujan*, edited by Vinay Dharwadker (Oxford: Oxford University Press, 1999), 134.
[255] Sathaye, Adheesh, ed. and trans. Forthcoming. Śivadāsa's *Twenty-Five Tales of the Vetāla.* Cambridge, MA: Harvard University Press.

which would include both elite and non-elite members of the court or of Brahmanical or monastic circles.[256]

The vetāla is found hanging from a tree in the *śmaśāna* (charnel grounds), and while it allows itself to get caught by the king, there are conditions. The vetāla tells a series of stories to the king, and towards the end of each story, he asks a riddle. The vetāla magically returns back to the tree if one speaks to it, so the stipulation is that if the king knows the answer but does not tell it, then his heart will burst and he will die. So, the king has to speak if he knows the answer. Thus, the only way for the king to succeed in taking the vetāla to the guru is if the king does not know the answer and so does not speak. Surprisingly, the guru turns out to be nefarious in that he will use the king's head and the vetāla's head in order to complete his sacrificial ritual to the goddess in order to acquire the siddhis (supernatural powers). Clearly, this is a set of tales that are not favorable towards tantrics, but since they are meant to be humorous, it is hard to extrapolate the impressions they leave about yoga practice and beliefs—let alone yogis themselves—to the feeling of the general population at the time.

I will examine three of the stories in the collection: story 17, "The Tale of the Tantric Goddess," story 21, "The Tale of Lion-Makers," and story 22, "Yogānanda's Tale."

The seventeenth story in Śivadāsa's compilation, "The Tale of the Tantric Goddess," is about a brahmin man who is addicted to gambling, is cast out of his home, and comes upon a yogi. The yogi offers him food from a skull but since he is a brahmin, he will not eat from it. The yogi uses his tantric powers to call upon a *yakṣiṇī* (female nature spirit) who gives the brahmin anything he wants for the night and when he wakes the next morning she is gone. He is desperate to find her and asks the yogi how to call her. The yogi teaches him the rituals, but they fail, and

[256] Sathaye, "How the Guru Lost His Power," 27. See also Adheesh Sathaye, "The Scribal Life of Folktales in Medieval India," *South Asian History and Culture* 8, no. 4 (2017), 435.

when the yogi tries again himself, he also fails, because the yakṣiṇī thinks the yogi taught someone undeserving so is no longer worthy himself. An extensive analysis of this story, in all four major versions of the VP, is found in Sathaye (2022).

The twenty-first story, titled "The Tale of Lion-Makers," is a tale of four brothers who were troubled. One was a gambler, one enjoyed escorts, one slept with other men's wives, and the last was an atheist. To sort them out, their father decided to educate them. Realizing they lacked knowledge, the brothers set off to find teachers, and eventually reunited with newfound tantric abilities. Ultimately, they were able to resurrect a lion using magic and the lion, once alive, ate the brothers. The implication is that having knowledge via an acquisition of yogic powers is not enough—one must also have intelligence.

In the twenty-second story, "Yogānanda's Tale," a brahmin spends his lifetime perfecting the yogic art of switching bodies. When he becomes old and weak, he decides to use this knowledge to acquire a young body. He goes to the cremation ground and finds the body of a young boy, into whose corpse he transfers his consciousness. Upon leaving his old body, he cries, and upon entering the new one, he laughs. The vetāla asks the king why the brahmin laughs and cries, and the king answers that as he was leaving the old body, he remembered how his parents had cared for his old body and how much he had enjoyed it in his youth, thus he cries; as he enters the new body, he laughs because he is young again— implying that he is going to get to enjoy all pleasures again.

These are depictions of yogis we have not really seen in the literature yet, though the PYS, and other primary yoga texts, deals extensively with siddhis. There was some hint in the PC of yoga practice giving people supernatural powers, such as in verse 14 of Act 3 when the Kāpālika lists the ways he can manipulate the elements, such as flooding the earth, but it was not quite as explicit as it is here, as the Kāpālika is never called a yogi. In the PC, the Kāpālika suggests the abilities are because of the gods, being able to call upon them at will. In the VP, the yogi is described as gaining the ability to switch bodies because of their own lifelong practice and dedication to it. The KS did not really consider magical abilities as any focal point to yogic practice. But here, we see that yogis are defined as people who practice to achieve magical powers, with even more emphasis than the yogic goal of liberation. There could be two reasons for this depiction. First, the author is making fun of the yogis and not taking their goals or practice seriously. Second, there was more tantric influence in the religious milieu at the time that was noticed by the people's perception of yogis and their practices.

These two options are not mutually exclusive, and as we saw earlier, tantrism was shifting its focus from asceticism to supernatural power. This is also evident of the larger shift from the PYS-era perception that the body is impure, to the body being a tool that can be used for self-oriented worldly goals rather than explicitly discarded. The transition represents the shift in the public idea that tantric practitioners were not only interested in sensual pleasures but also rather addicted to them. This also reflects a kind of jealousy by the public that the tantric and yogic practitioners desire the same things as the general public but because of their powers, they can potentially get what they want more easily. We see this in the seventeenth story where the brahmin learns tantric rituals in order to achieve the worldly pleasures the yakṣiṇī provides, despite his family saying he can have all the happiness at home. We also saw evidence of this in the PC when the Kāpālika was freely sexual, partaking in alcohol and drugs, and generally hedonistic.

The yogis in these stories look like typical ascetics: dirty, matted hair, emaciated, wearing little-to-no clothing or uncomfortable clothing, living in the elements with no food or water other than what was given to them, and seated in extended periods of meditation. This imagery is not new, nor has it seemingly evolved from the time of Kālidāsa and his extensive description of Pārvatī's tapasyā. What has changed most about the descriptions is that they are shown to lack the magical- or will-powers that they claim to have, or at least to be able to utilize them effectively and maintain them. Since this is roughly contemporary with the PC, it is not surprising that we see similar depictions there, even though they are most likely talking about two different groups of people; the PC was talking about Kāpālikas and the VP is talking about an unnamed array of yogis, which frankly could be from any number of traditions, or simply ascetics unaffiliated with a particular school. The yogi in story 17 does offer food out of his skull-bowl, which is a sign of being a Kāpālika, but not all the stories are that explicit. These yogis in the VP seem to be generic stand-ins for anyone who might fit the description, leaving it up to the audience to determine for themselves who specifically it represents. This is a key aspect of the incongruity theory of humour wherein the subject is not explicit, but rather is pointed at in the assumption that either the audience will understand the context and know who or what is being referred to, or the audience will be able to map their own ideas of what that reference is supposed to be which allows it to be many things at once.[257]

While the VP does not reveal new details about how yoga practitioners went about the pursuit of yoga, or about the intricacies of yoga as a philosophy, this text, by lampooning the yogic practitioner, reflects public anxieties about the validity of their practices and abilities, and the impact that may have on society as a whole, as well as each individual. It does not actively address yogic beliefs or describe yoga practices in any great detail but is important for the sake

[257] Qiaoyun Chen and Guiying Jiang, "Why are you amused: Unveiling multimodal humor from the prototype theoretical perspective," in *The European Journal of Humour Research* 6, no. 1 (June 2018). https://doi.org/10.7592/EJHR2018.6.1.chen

of understanding the public perception of yogis to be a primarily hesitant if not explicitly anxious.

Conclusions

In section 3, two of the four texts examined were explicitly satirical in their depictions of yogis and tantrics. I noted that one of the reasons for satire was, according to Sathaye (2022), so the audience could view these peripheral groups from a safe distance. I furthered that argument by stating the idea that there was some anxiety about the possible outcomes of partaking in such viewing or questioning in a more personal, non-satirical setting, such as confronting an actual practitioner.[258] To me, the need to confront these ideas through satire speaks to the fact that there was some cultural anxiety about whether or not these practitioners actually could do the things they claimed, and what implication that would have on the real world and the people in it. It also suggests an inferiority complex towards yogis wherein the public definitely cannot switch bodies or sleep with forest goddesses. But yogis can, or at least claim to, and so we are jealous, nervous about their powers, and also—importantly—voyeuristically interested in playing out the fantasy from a distance. Siegel (1987) claimed that "Satiric laughter is a medicine," and while that may be part of what is happening in the satire here—i.e., providing relief of the jealousy and anxiety—it seems to me that while these texts were clearly poking fun at the "others," they were also inherently lending some legitimacy to them. As I mentioned in 3.4, the PC ends up legitimizing these schools by accepting them as able to "battle" on the side of the good actors in the play—namely, the Vedic schools. This suggests that there is at least a fraction of legitimacy to the schools, even if ultimately they end up disjointed anyway. While Sathaye (2022) does not think the VP tales are actively "othering" yogis, seemingly because they are poking fun at almost all groups of people, I believe that in itself is helping define the groups as separate from each other—not necessarily calling out one in particular or establishing a hierarchy. Sathaye's (2017)

[258] For a more detailed examination of these anxieties, see Sathaye, "How the Guru Lost his Power," 11-12.

article explains that the scribes who copied Śivadāsa's VP were of quite the variety—brahmins, Kayastha, Jain, and probably others.[259] This variety suggests to me that each of these groups saw value in the tales, even though their beliefs and/or practices were mocked, which supports my idea of othering as a tool of categorization and comparison rather than promoting a Foucauldian hierarchy.

The satirical outcome of "othering" these groups in both the PC and VP hearkens to the topics discussed in section two, where al-Birūni was grappling with framing the narratives of the "other" through a more respectful lens than his predecessors. Incidentally, he was doing so in the same century as the PC and VP were composed, which shows that it was not just the Islamicate scholars interested in yoga or defining groups. Al-Birūni recognized that other scholars and writers were disregarding and demeaning what they did not understand—nor cared to understand. I argue that the satire we see in the PC is demeaning the "others" but not disregarding them, and VP is doing both, demeaning and/or disregarding them, though with more light-heartedness than we saw in the PC as this satire was not aimed at just one or a few groups—it is everybody. Al-Birūni was more accurate than he realized, for he was speaking about the scholars and writers he was familiar with—namely other Islamicate works—but the same applies for people already embedded in the Vedic and Hindu religious milieu. The difference, of course, is the degree of difference (or similarity, as it may be) between the Islamicate writers and yogis, and the Sanskrit writers and yogis. The Sanskrit writers were in a sense moving away from the yogic religious groups, ideologically speaking, while the Islamicate writers were moving towards them, both literally and ideologically, as Sufi ideas became more pronounced, as examined in section two.

---

[259] Sathaye, "The Scribal Life of Folktales in Medieval India," 435.

Indeed, it seems that as the schools of belief of yoga and tantrism progressed, becoming more defined over time, the public's reaction become more alarmed. In the first two thirds of the first millennium BCE, Sanskrit writers were willing to engage with the ideas and practices with some sort of familiarity and as an exercise in understanding and adoption. But by the turn of the millennium, writers—and, if we can presume to extend it, the public—found the practices more alien, more transgressive, and thus were less willing to engage with them directly and so used the indirect route of satire to make them approachable.

This evolution is also seen in the primary texts as examined in the first section. The PYS was radical for its time but compared to the medieval tantric-influenced yoga practices it had a relatively Vedic flavour. Evidence was also shown that the PYS was influenced by Buddhism and seemed to be in conversation with the Buddhist texts, the *Upaniṣads*, and the *Vedas*, not to mention the Vaiśeṣika and Sāṃkhya philosophies, as they were grappling to understand the world. As both the primary and secondary texts show, the schools seemed to evolve away from each other until they were different enough that the Sanskrit literary authors felt they could only really deal with them in a satirical fashion. Importantly, it is not just the philosophies that the secondary literature is dealing with, but the yogis and practices themselves, which shows that it is likely that yoga practitioners were actively practicing what the treatises taught, even as they got more extreme and transgressive, which supplemented the public's anxieties. We do not see the same kind of satire in the Islamicate texts, though of course the "Medieval Sufi Tales of Jogis" compiled by Simon Digby were more along the same lines of making fun of yogis and has a similar feeling to the VP. This suggests that the Sufis were not as anxious about the way the yogis looked or what they practiced as the Sanskrit writers were, though of course the Sufis were critical of the yogic beliefs.

It would be interesting to examine later Sanskrit texts to see if the public perception about these schools shifted to be more inclusive again. We saw in the sixteenth-century Persian *Madhumālatī* a seemingly complete acceptance of yogic ascetic practice, if not belief, that I wonder if it existed in Sanskrit texts at the time as well. The general theme we can use to compare the Islamicate versus Sanskrit texts is metaphorical distancing. Muslim writers were already distanced from the yogis, while Brahmanical writers felt the need to create a certain distancing within the poetic descriptions—whether this is through literary devices like we saw with Kālidāsa and Māgha, or through irony and satire, as in the case of Kṛṣṇamiśra and Śivadāsa. Both Islamicate and Sanskrit writers all distanced themselves from their object of curiosity, the yogi, but for the Sanskrit writers this requires taking recourse to the tools of poetics, theatre, and storytelling.

Overall, it is not entirely possible to glean the public's perception of a group of practices and beliefs based on just eight texts, but it is a start that sheds light on the dynamics in the society at play. The anxieties, curiosities, and evolution of practices and beliefs is clear even in the literature, and it shows us that the primary texts were probably—in general—written about practices that were happening, rather than being written to start new practices. In other words, the changes were happening "on the ground," so to speak, rather than being pushed forward in writing. This appears to be a general trend in South Asian history, where literature and texts tended to be oral before they were written, meaning that the treatises followed the practices. It would be useful to compare this phenomenon to other cultures around the world to see if the religious and practical treatises tended to initiate evolutions in the practices or if the evolution spurred the writing of the texts. While this thesis is just a tiny fraction of the research that can contribute to this larger examination, I hope it is at least sufficient as a place to start.